ADULT COLORING BOOK

CIRCULAR PATTERNS

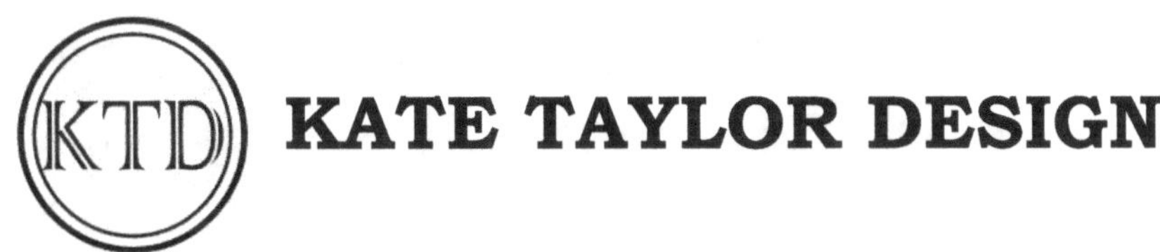

Adult coloring book, CIRCULAR PATTERNS presents 50 beautiful models that have been designed from simple shapes that are reflected on different axes of symmetry that converge to the center.

If you would like to reorder, please scan the QR Code

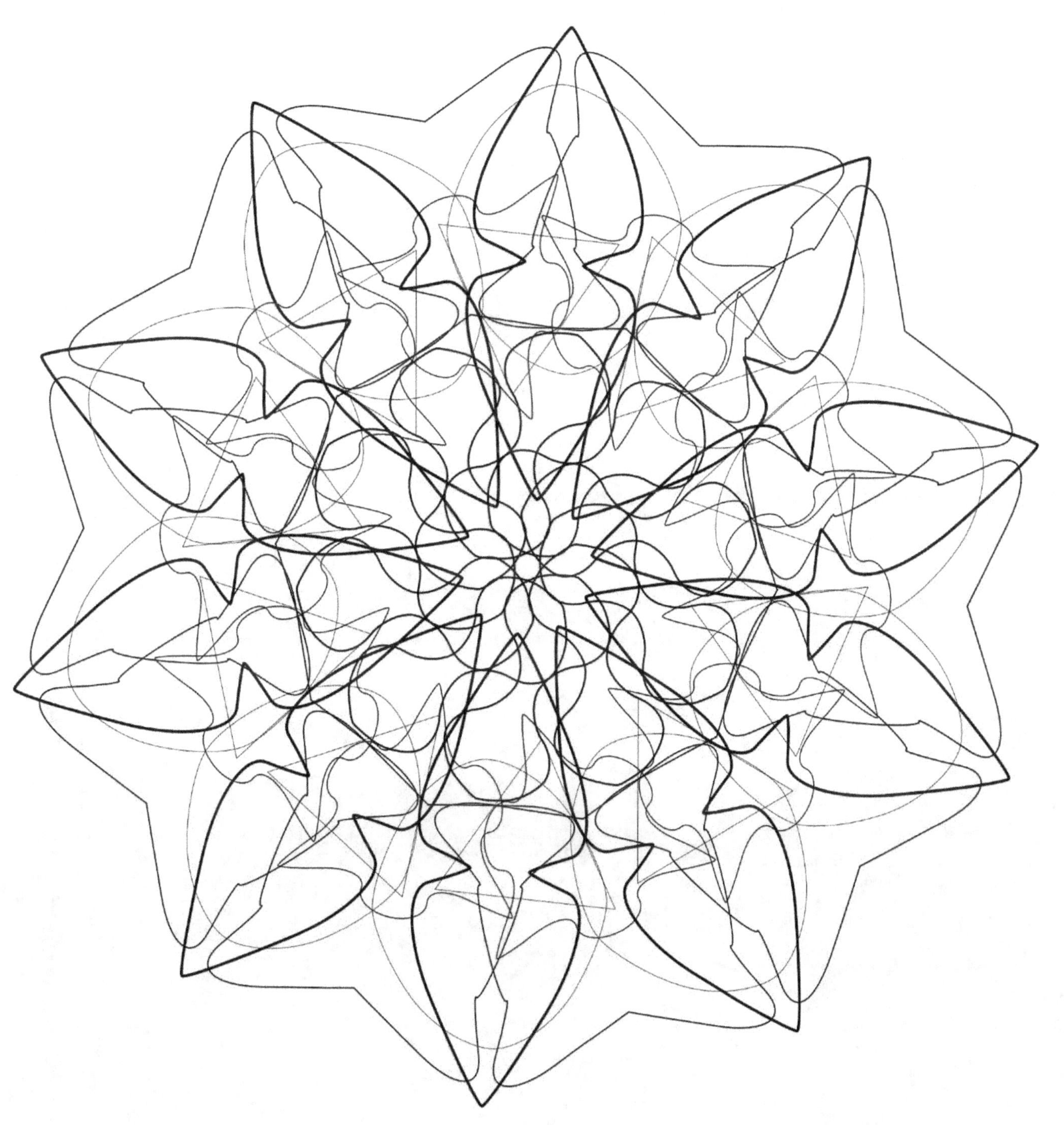

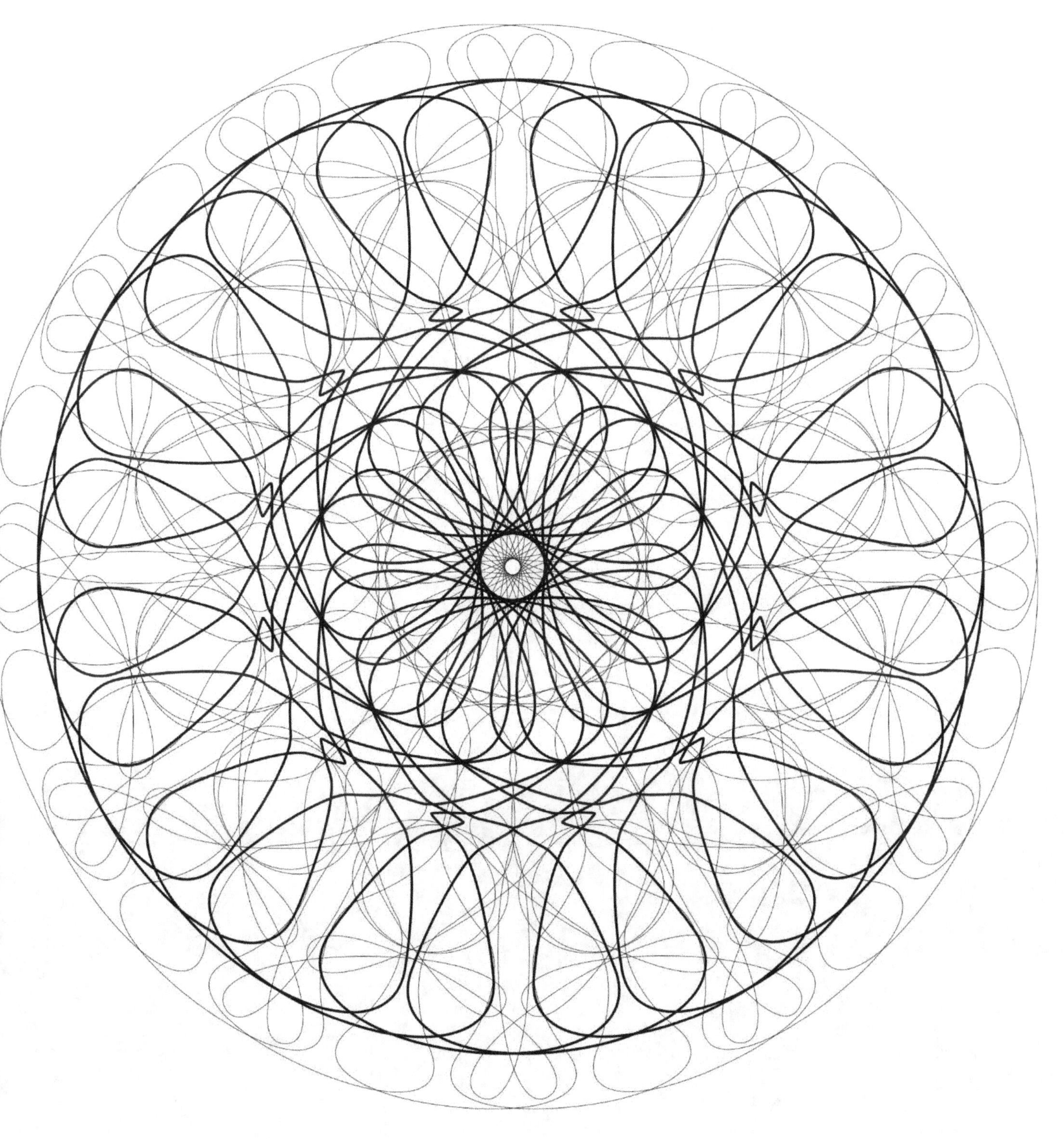

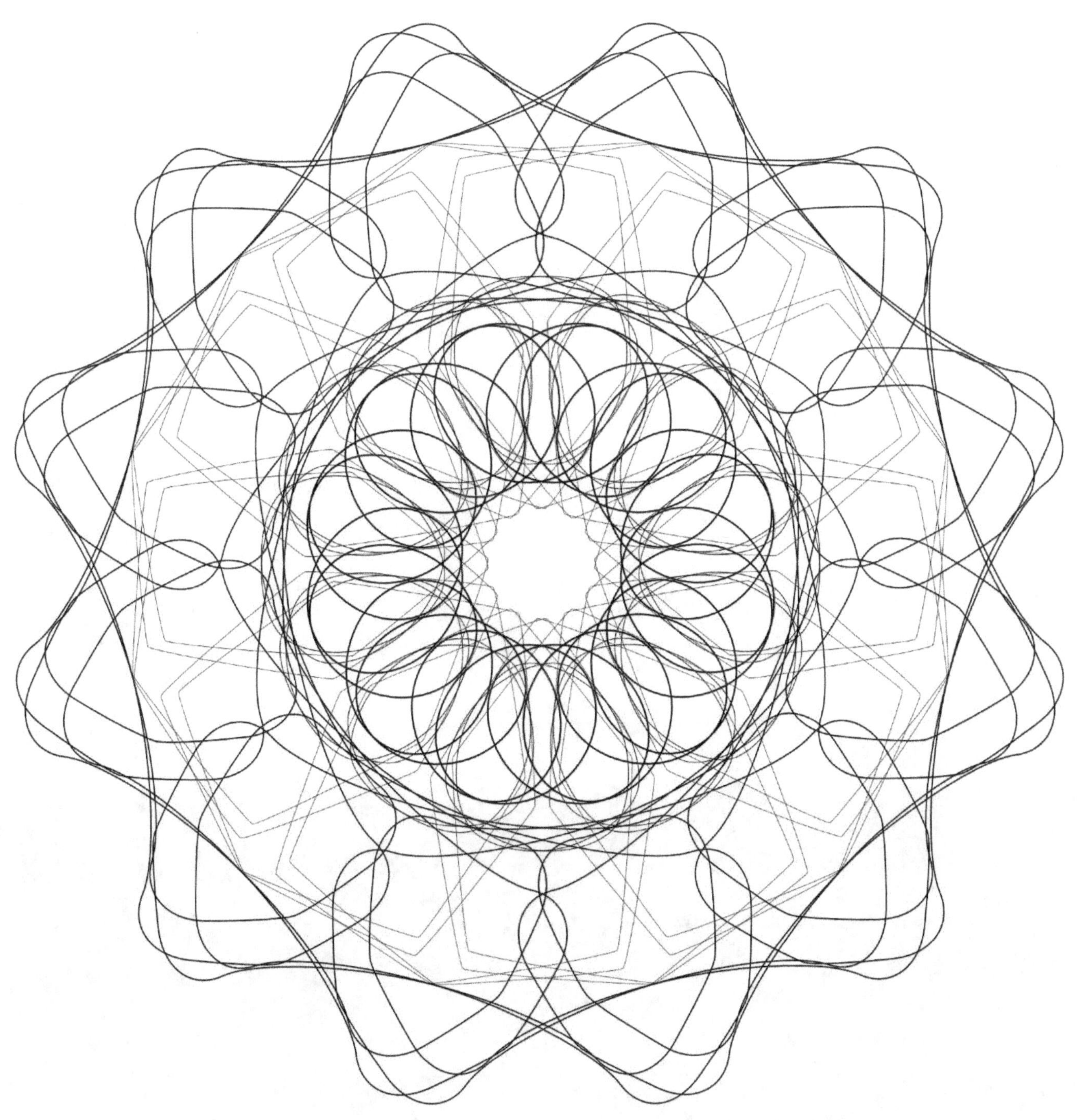

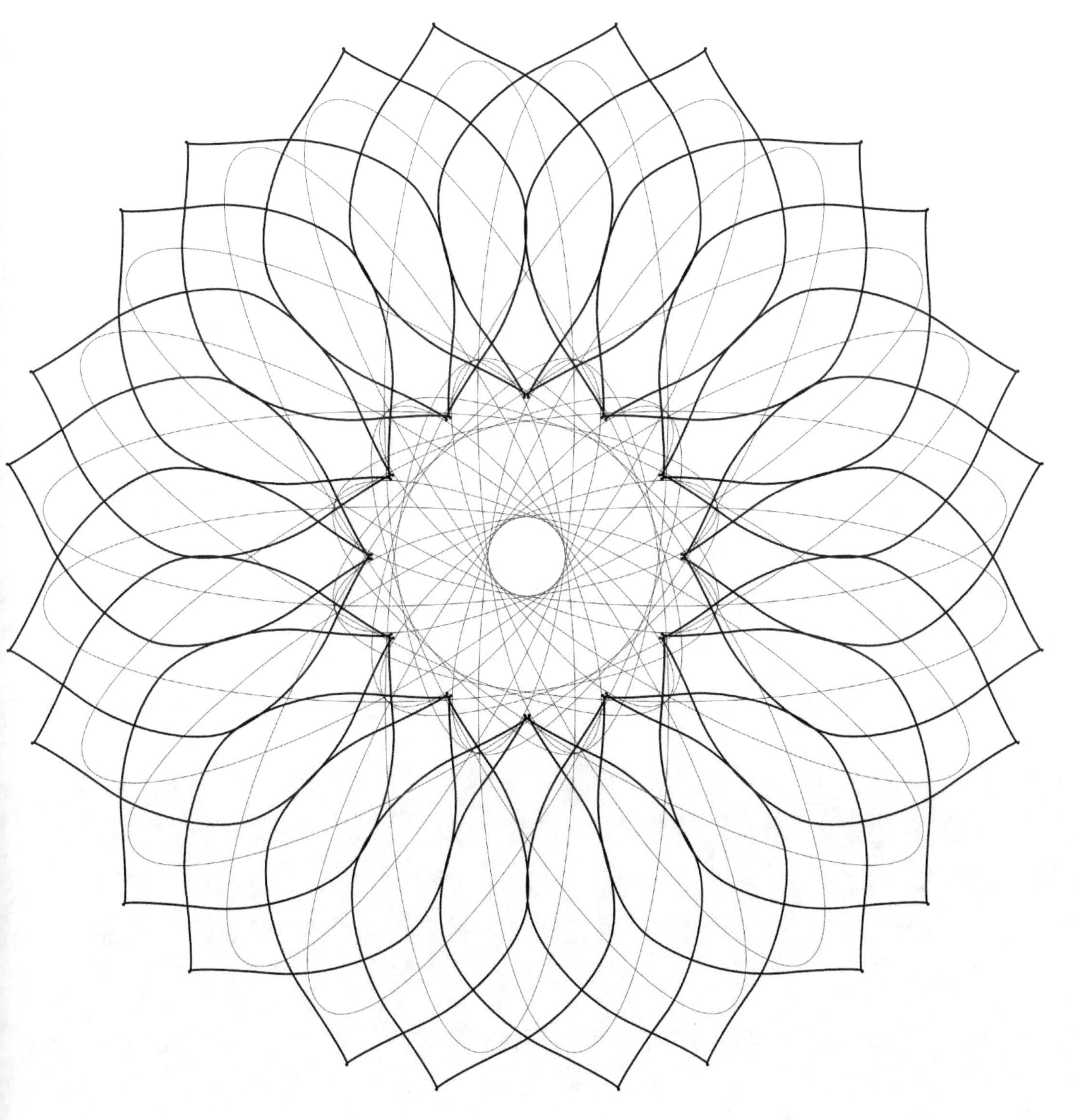

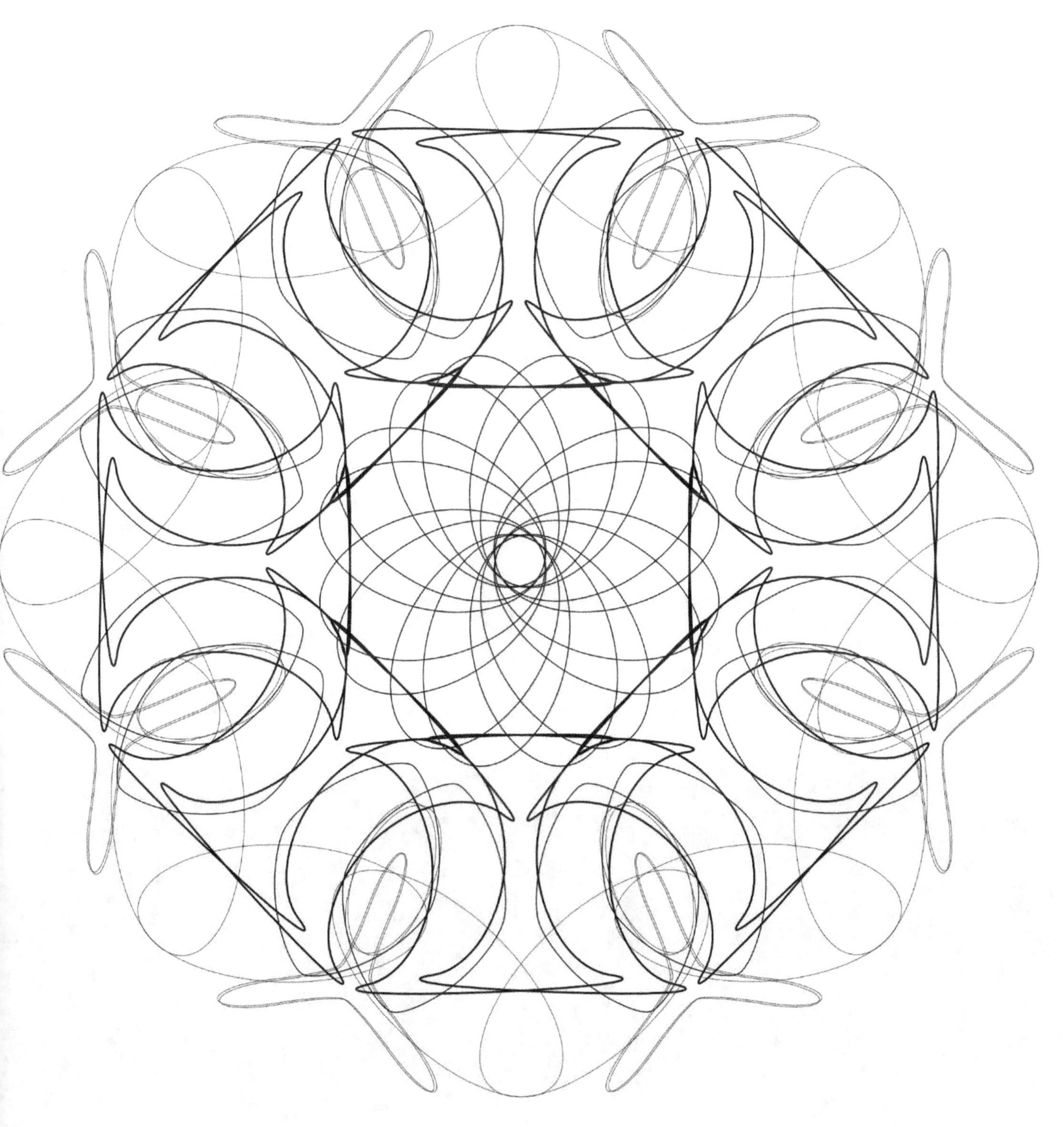

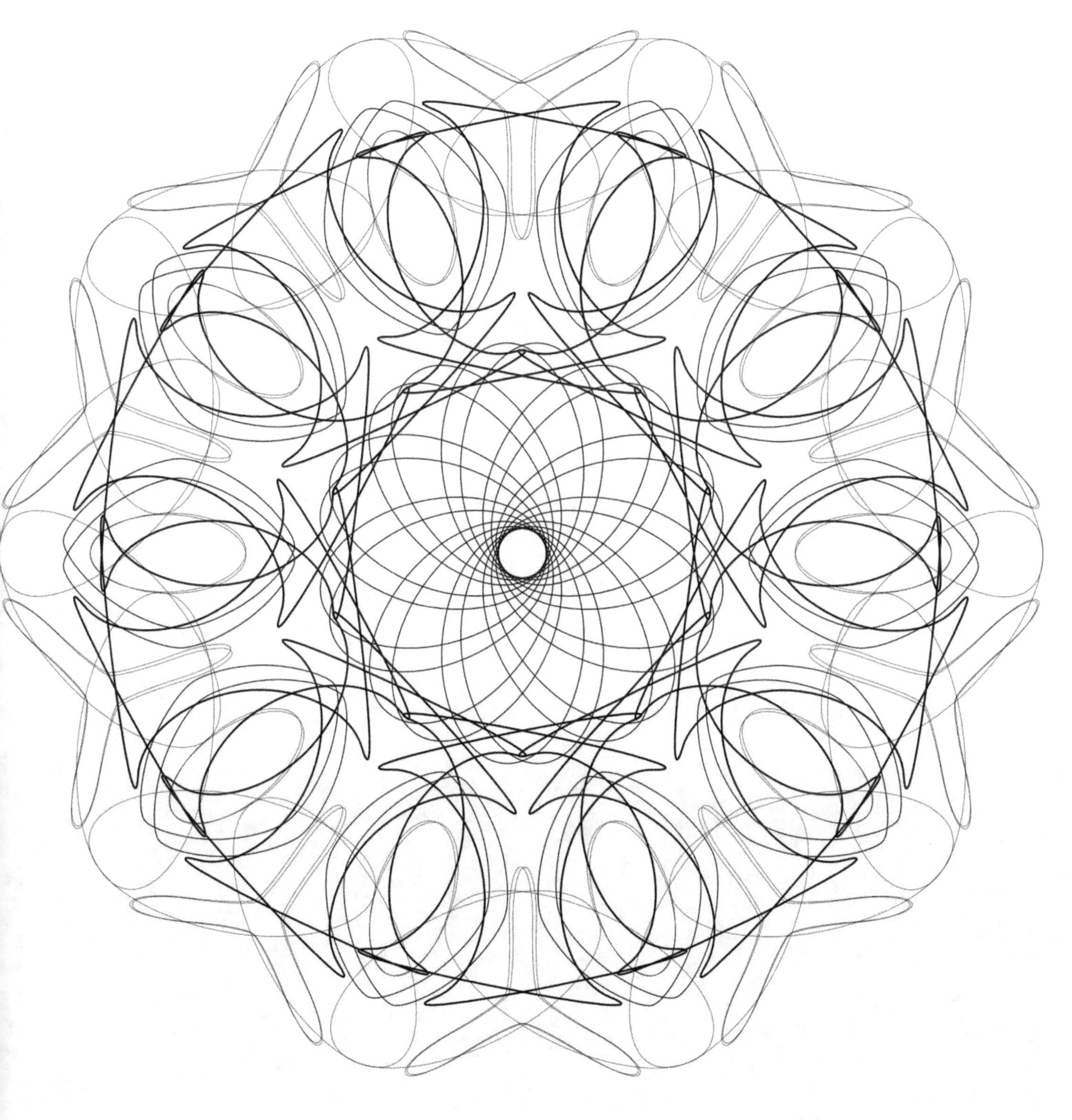

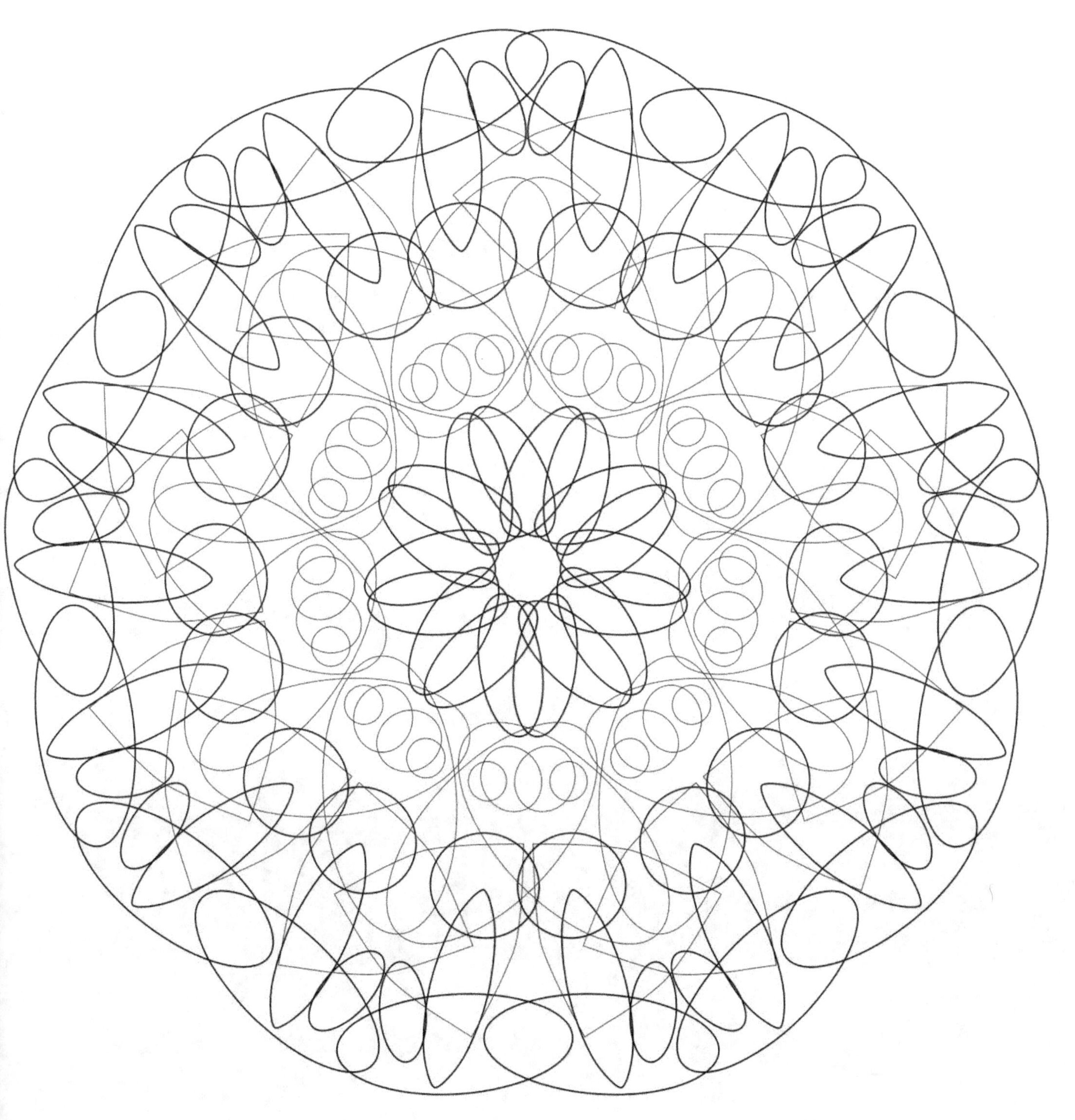

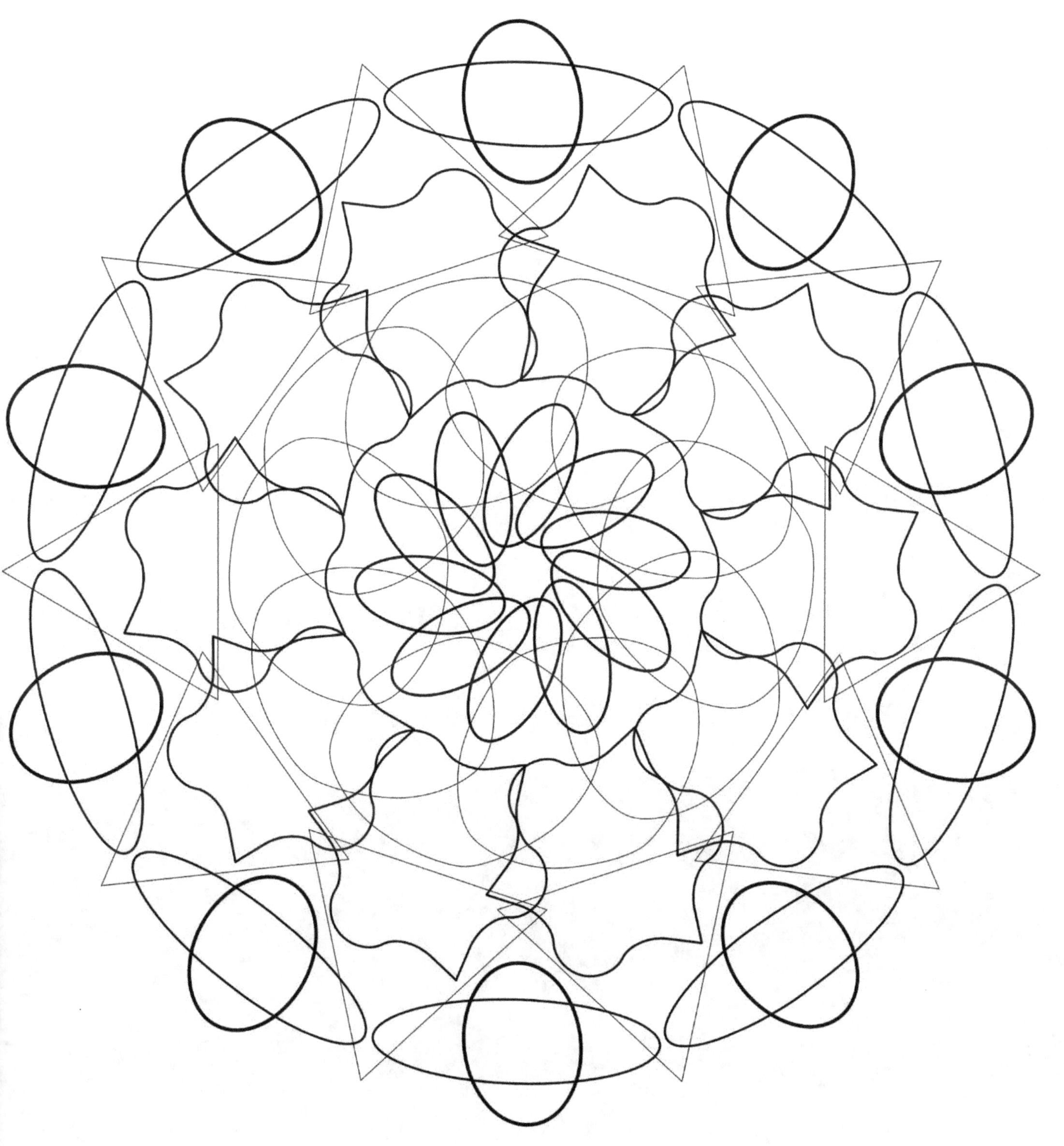

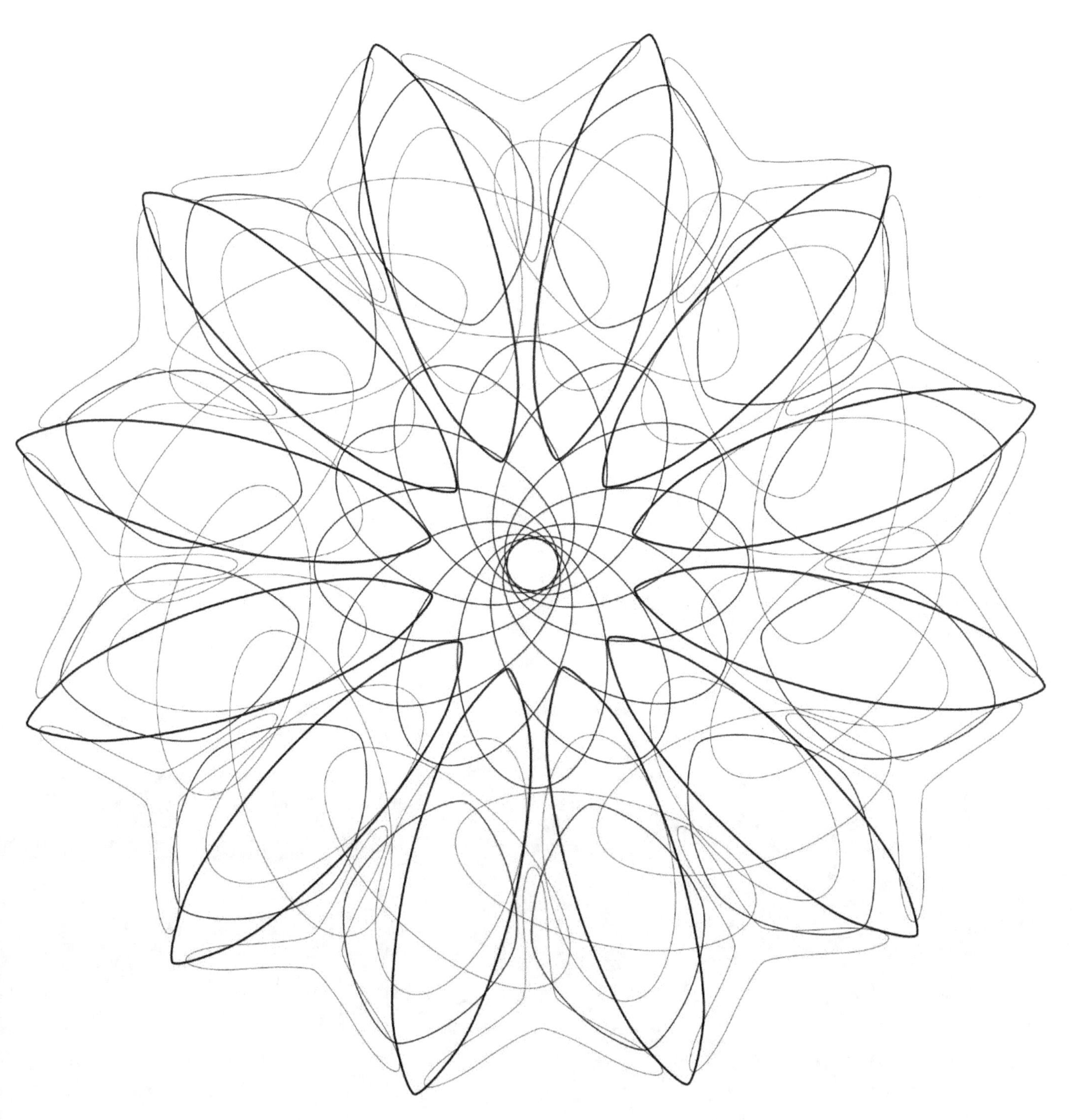

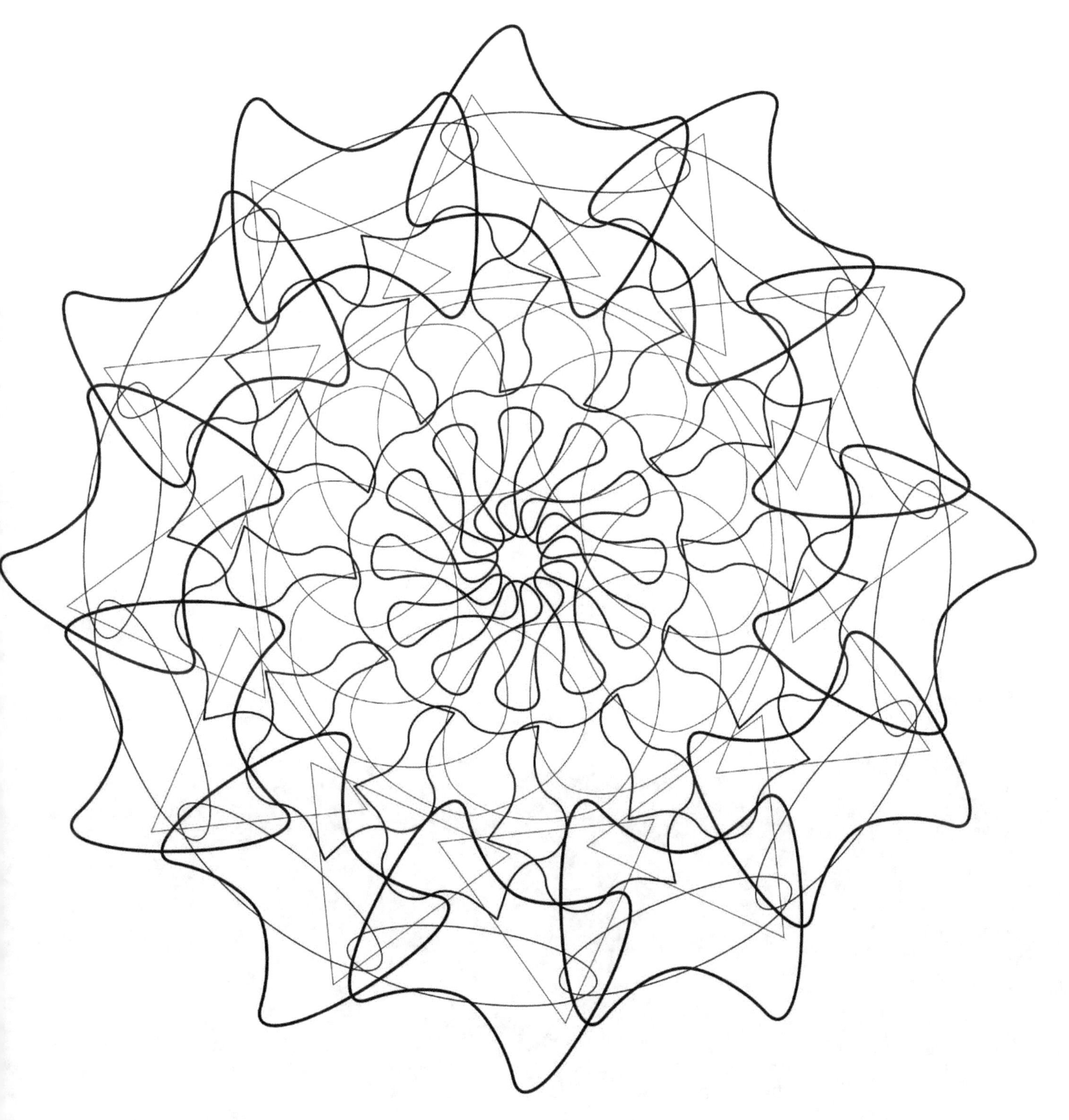

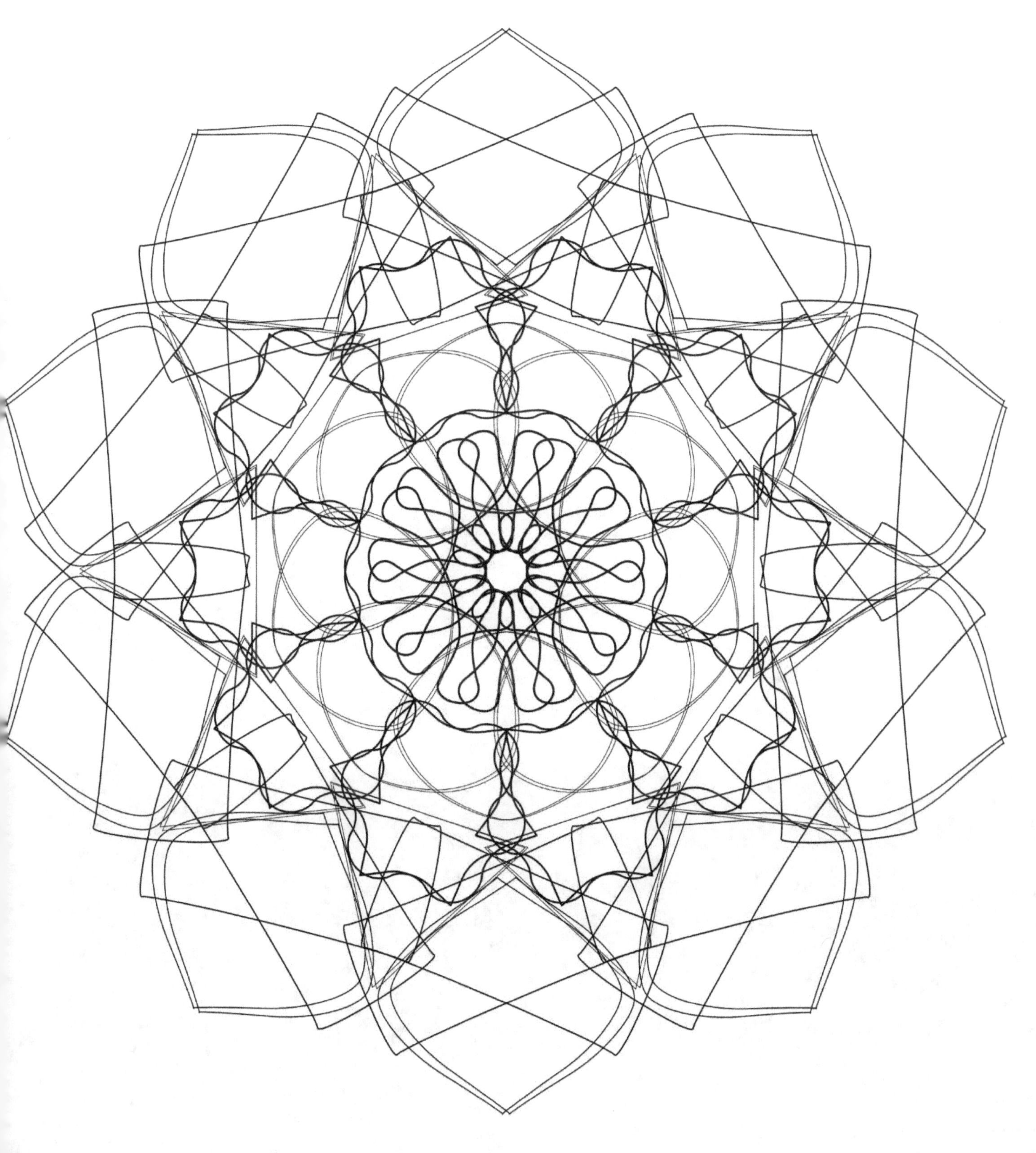

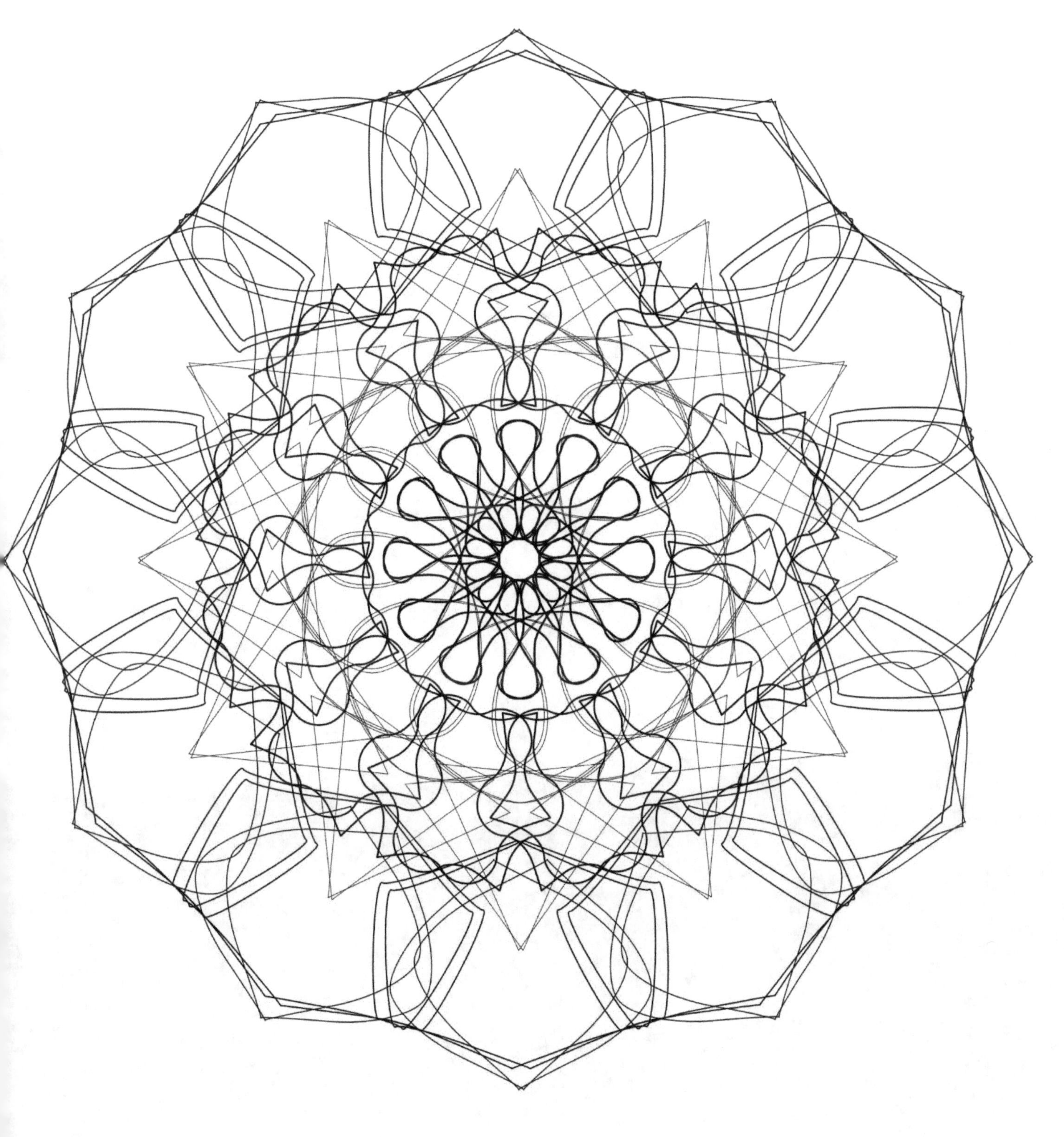

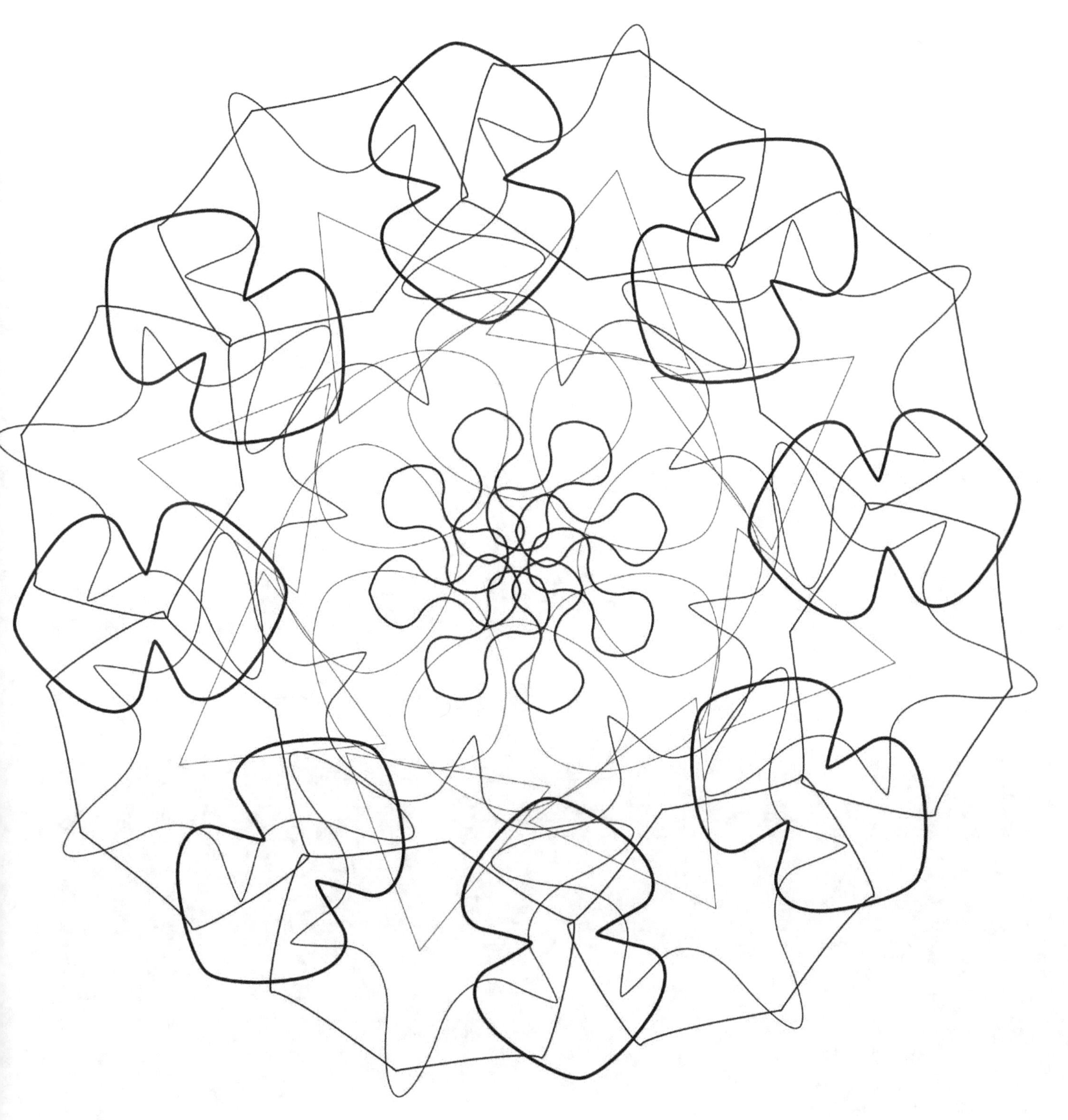

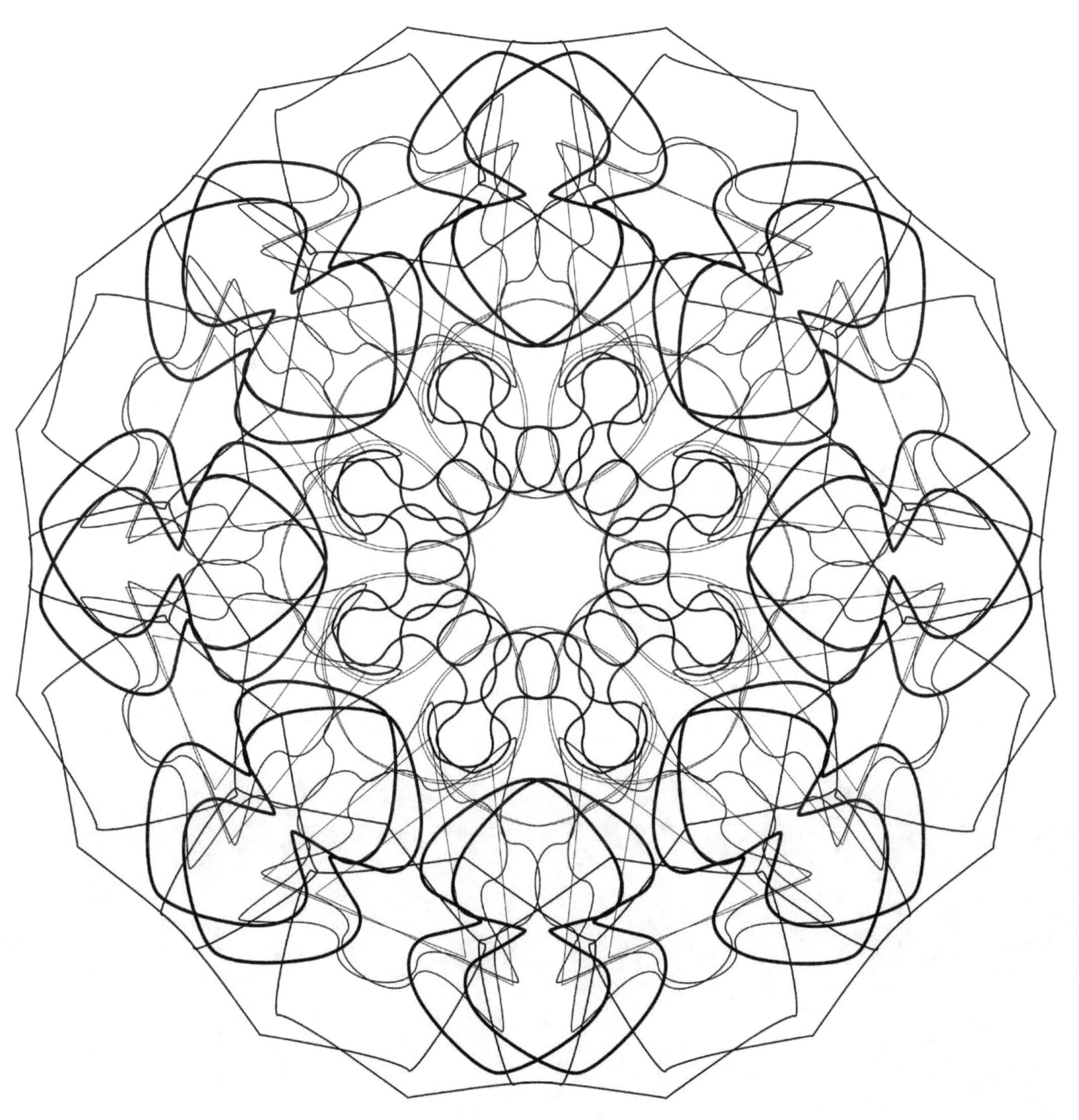

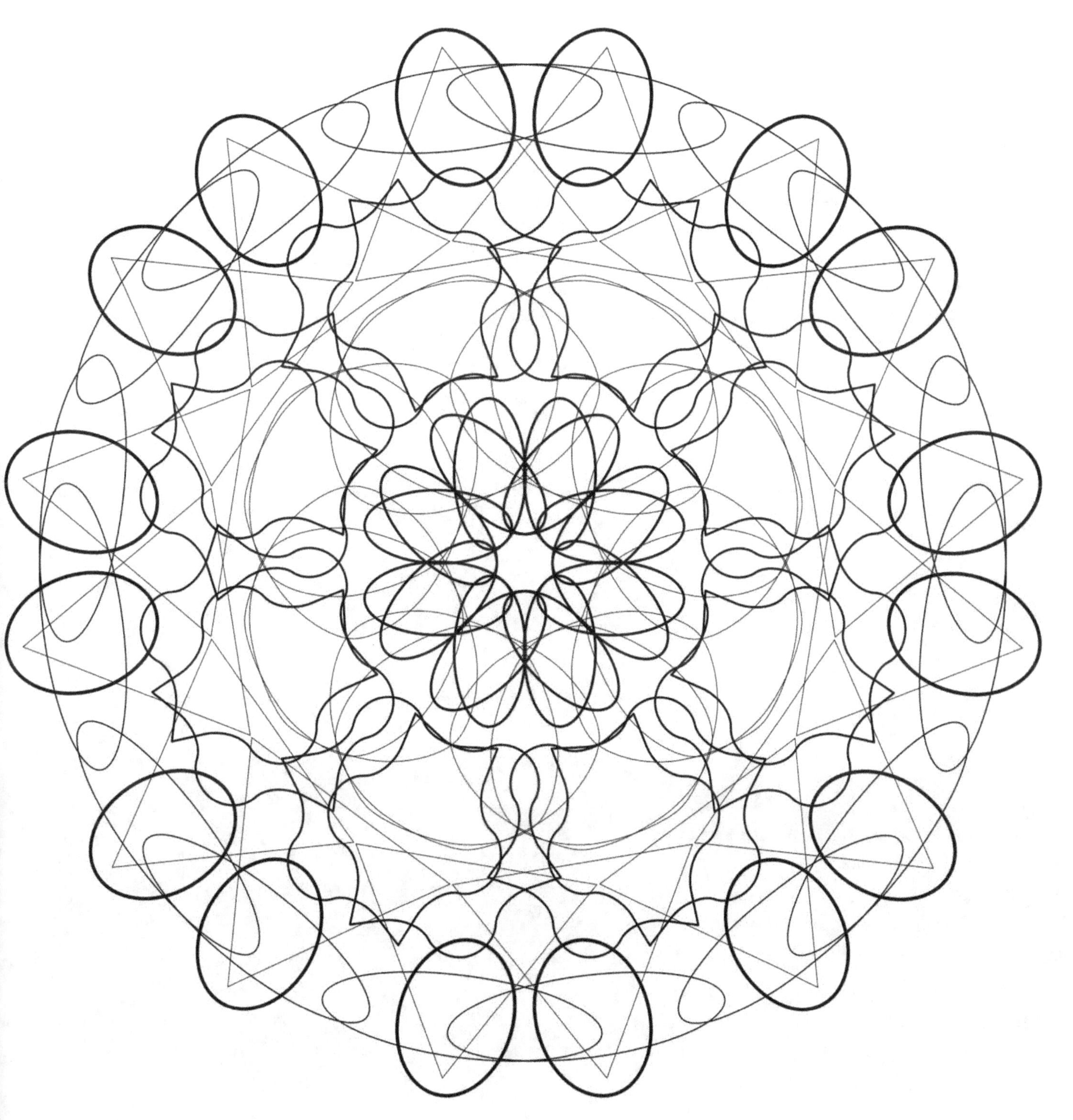

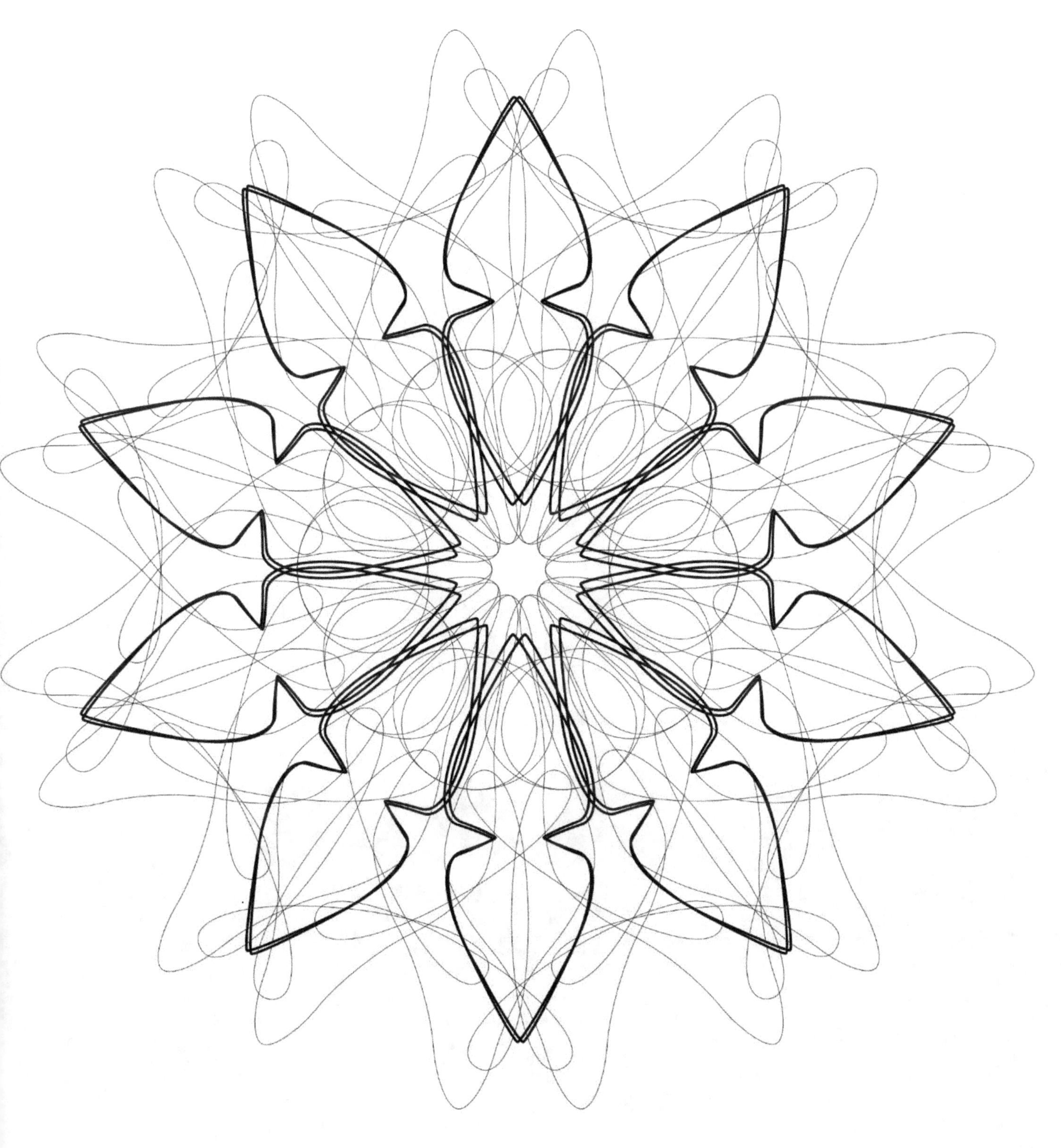

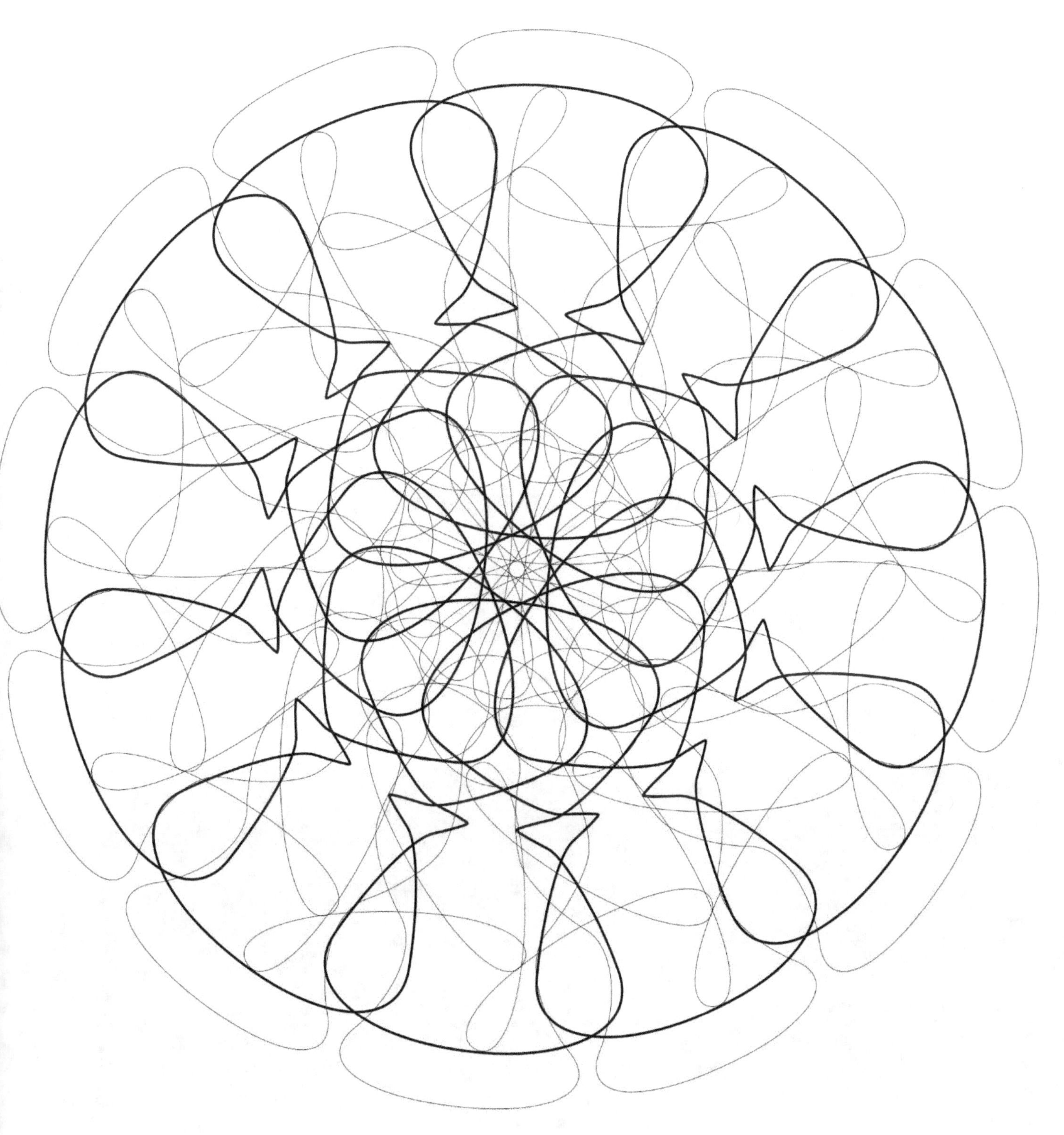

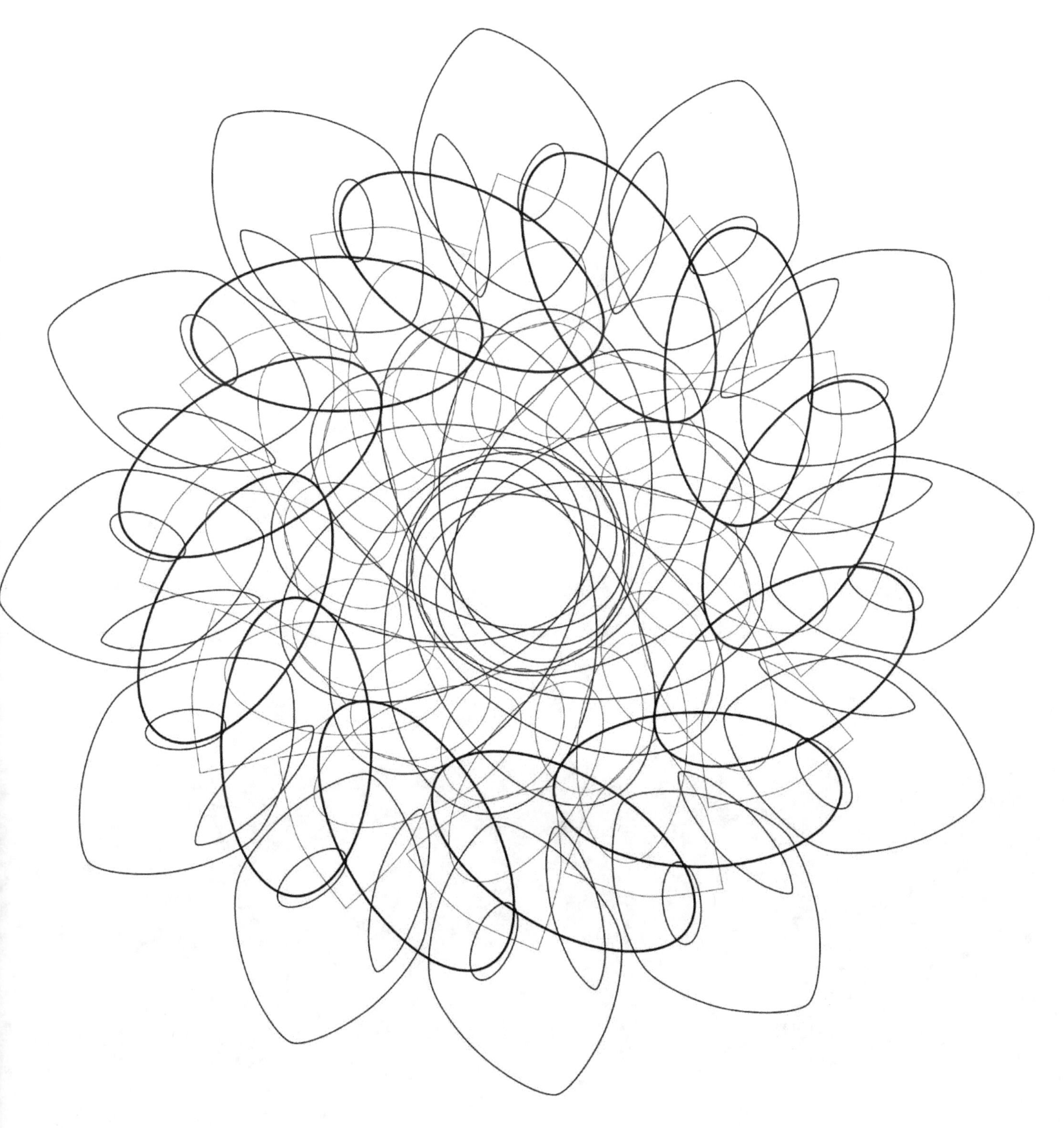

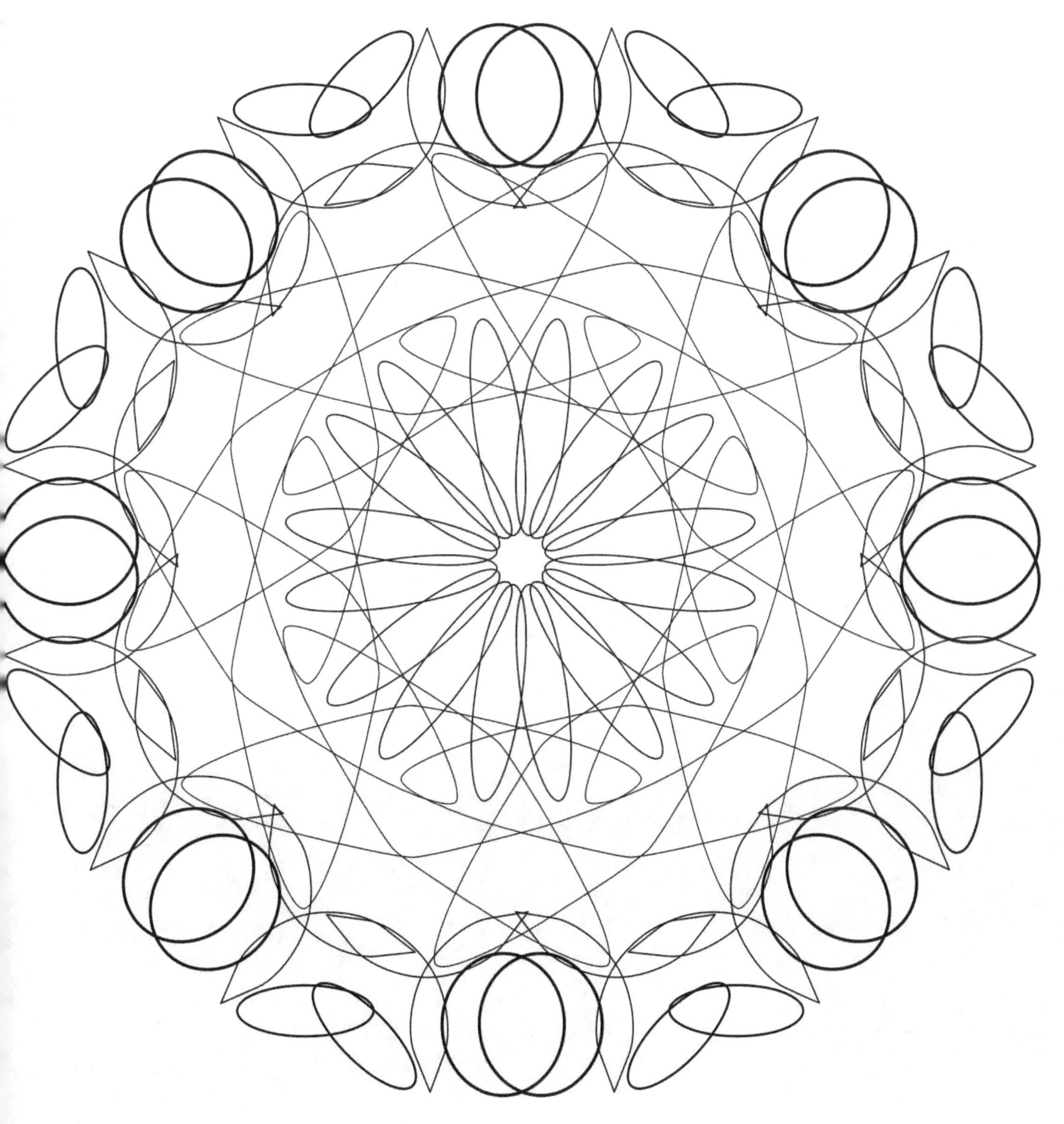

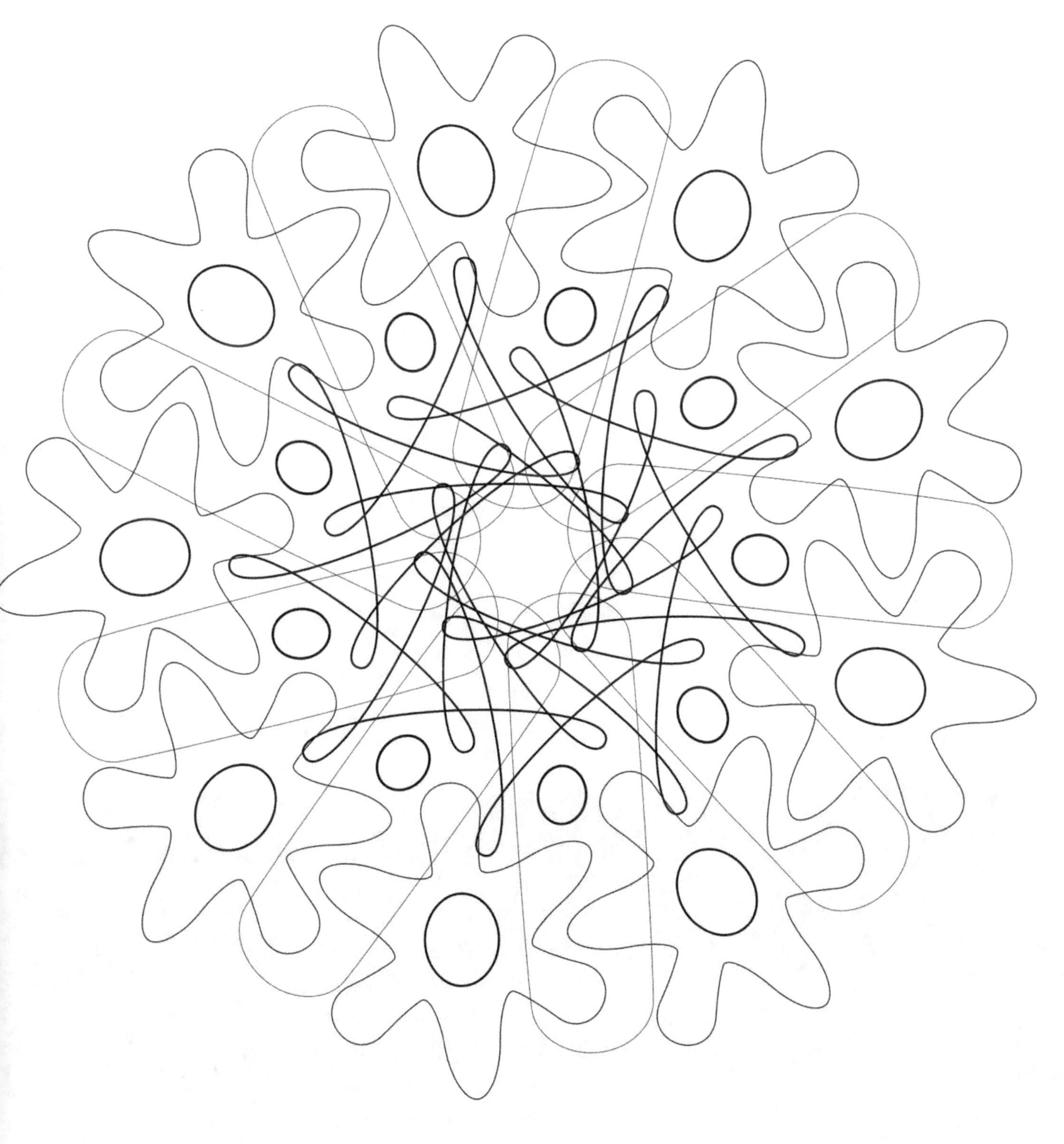

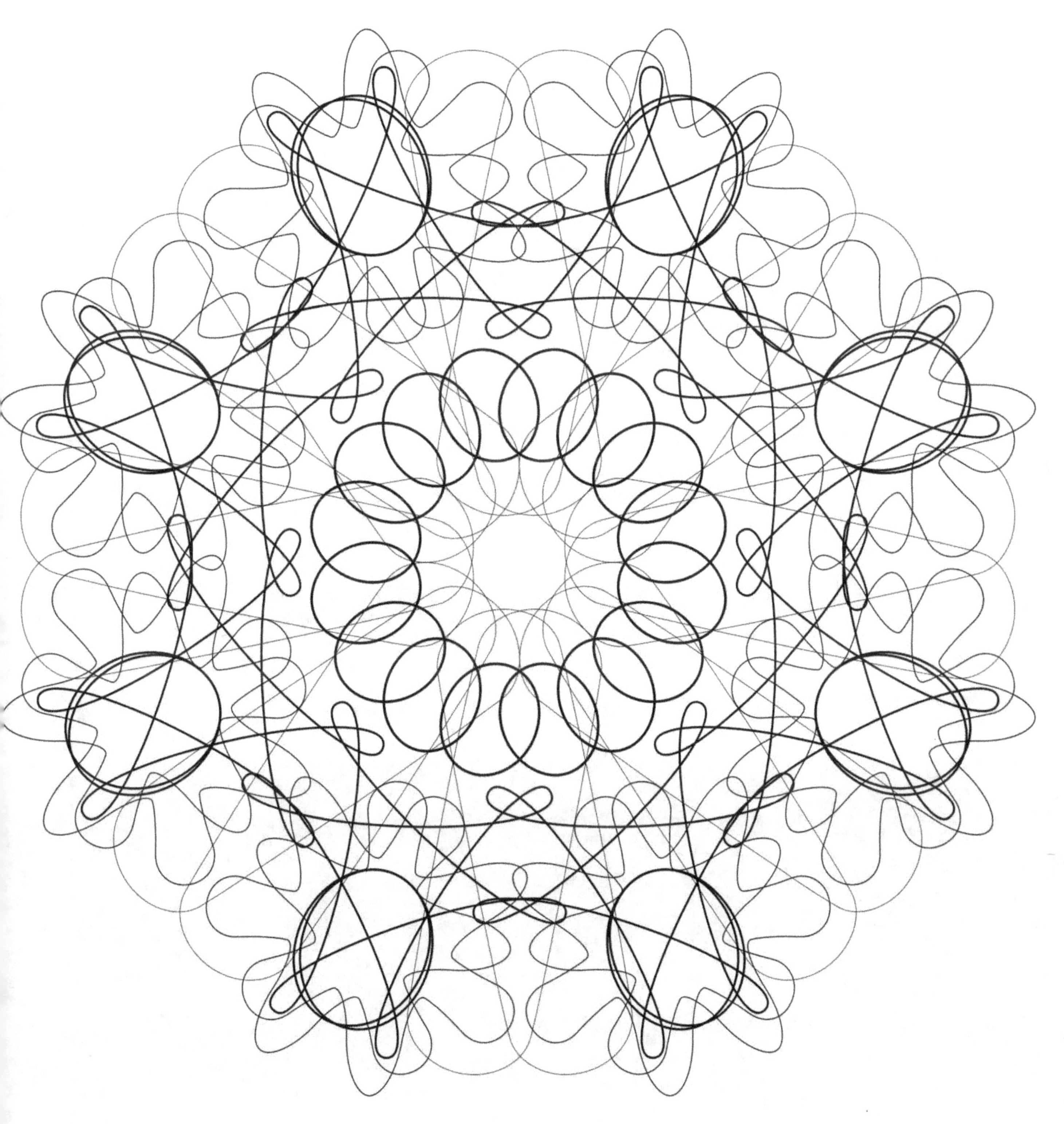

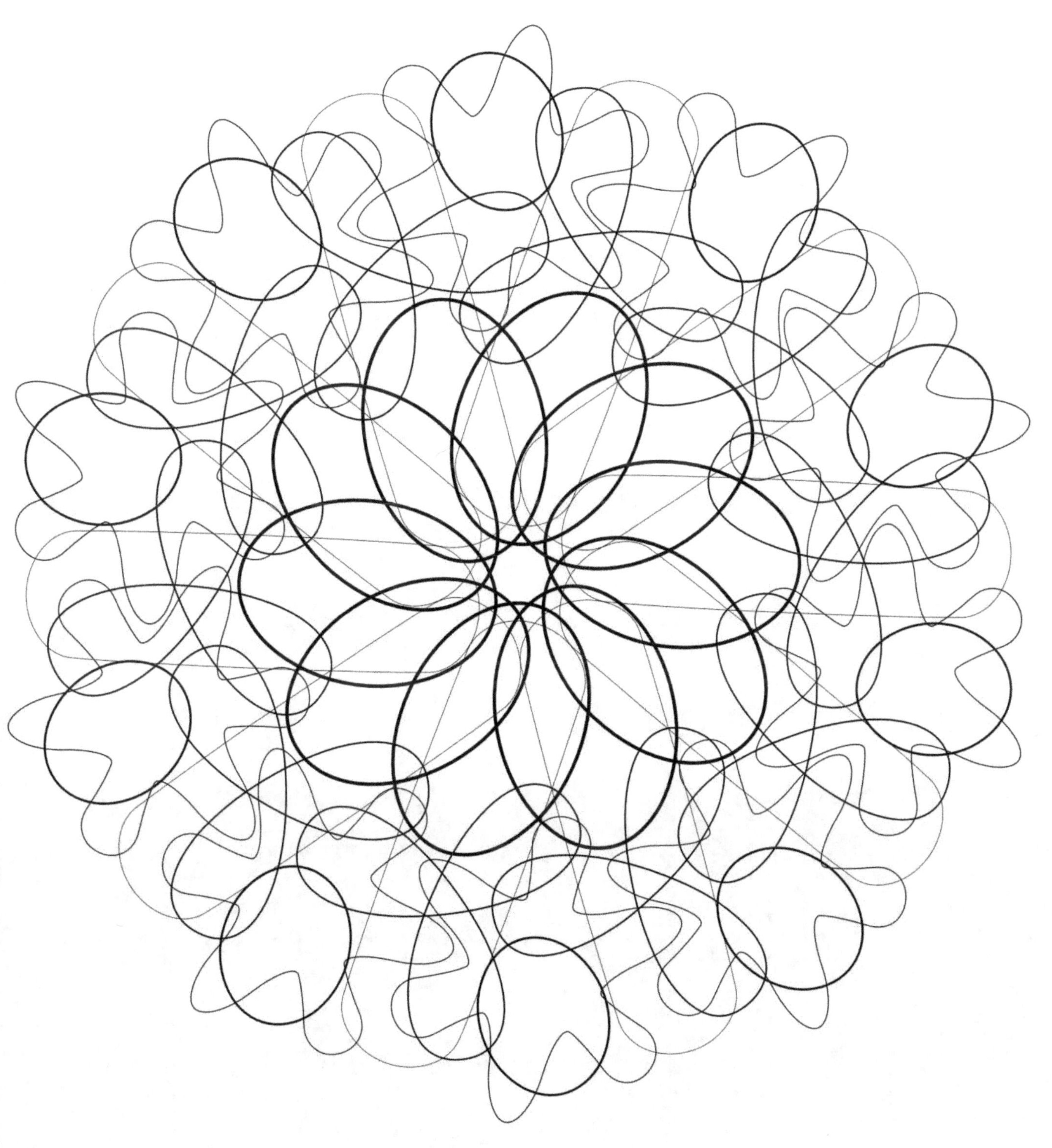

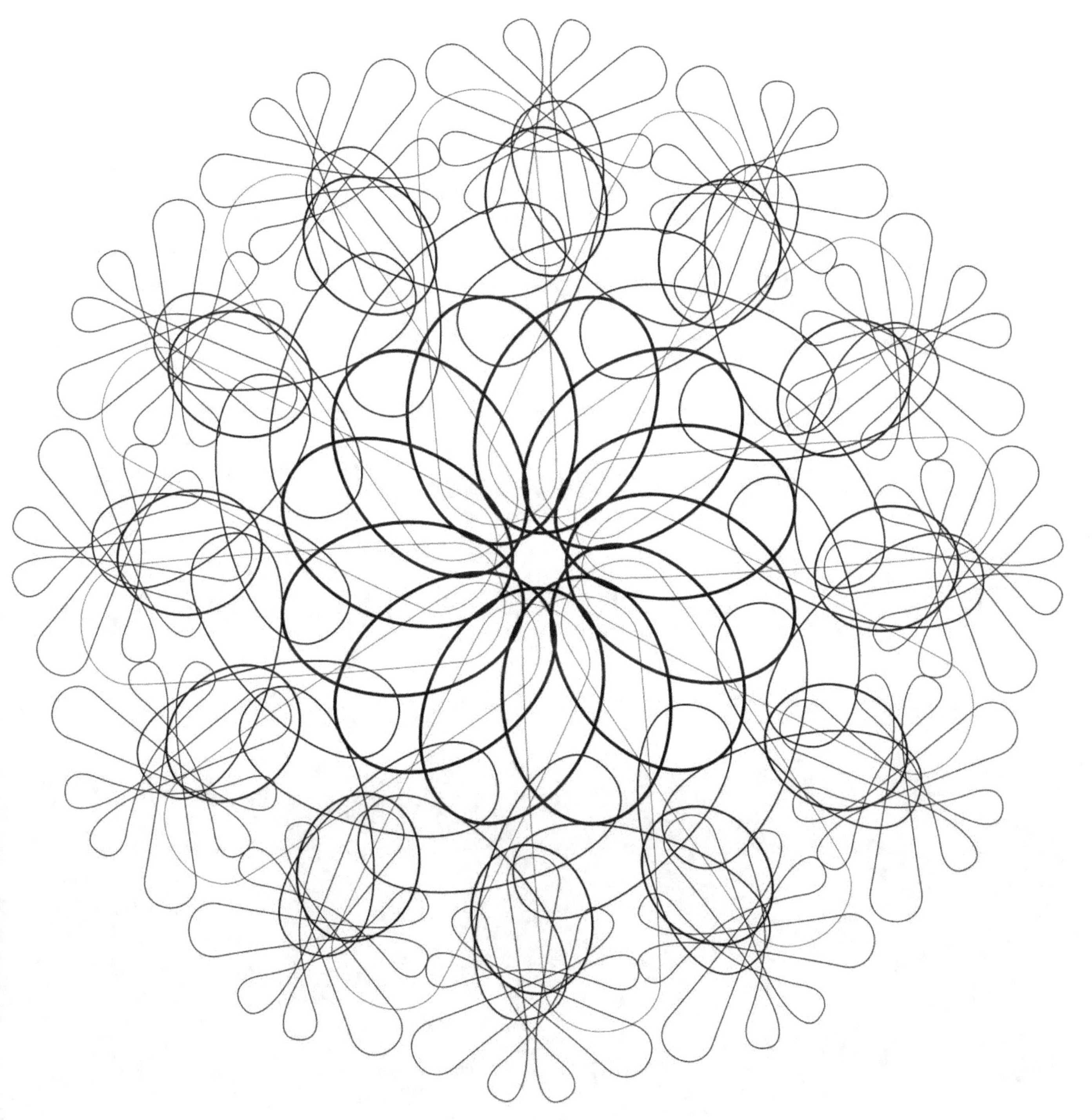

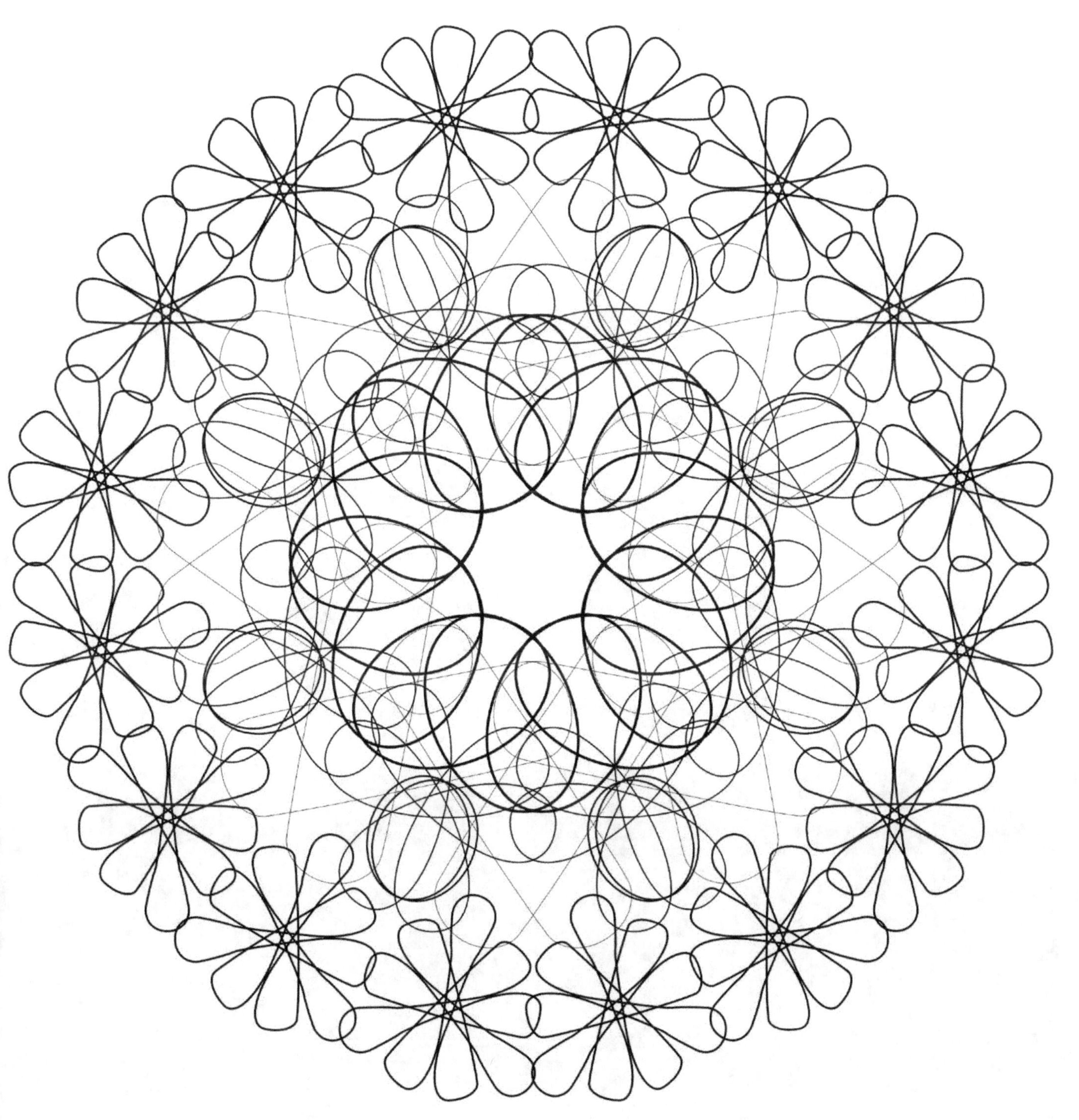

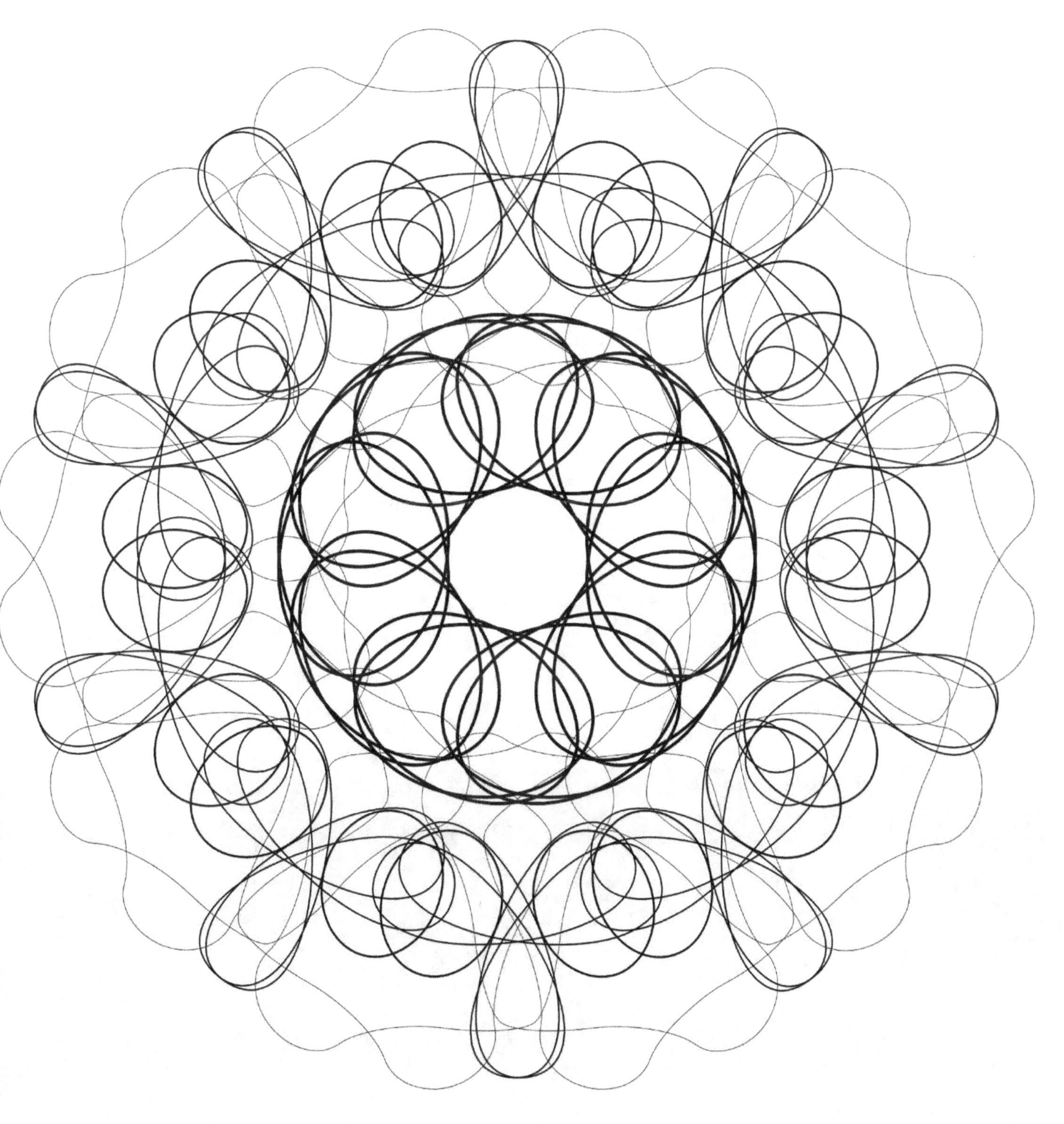

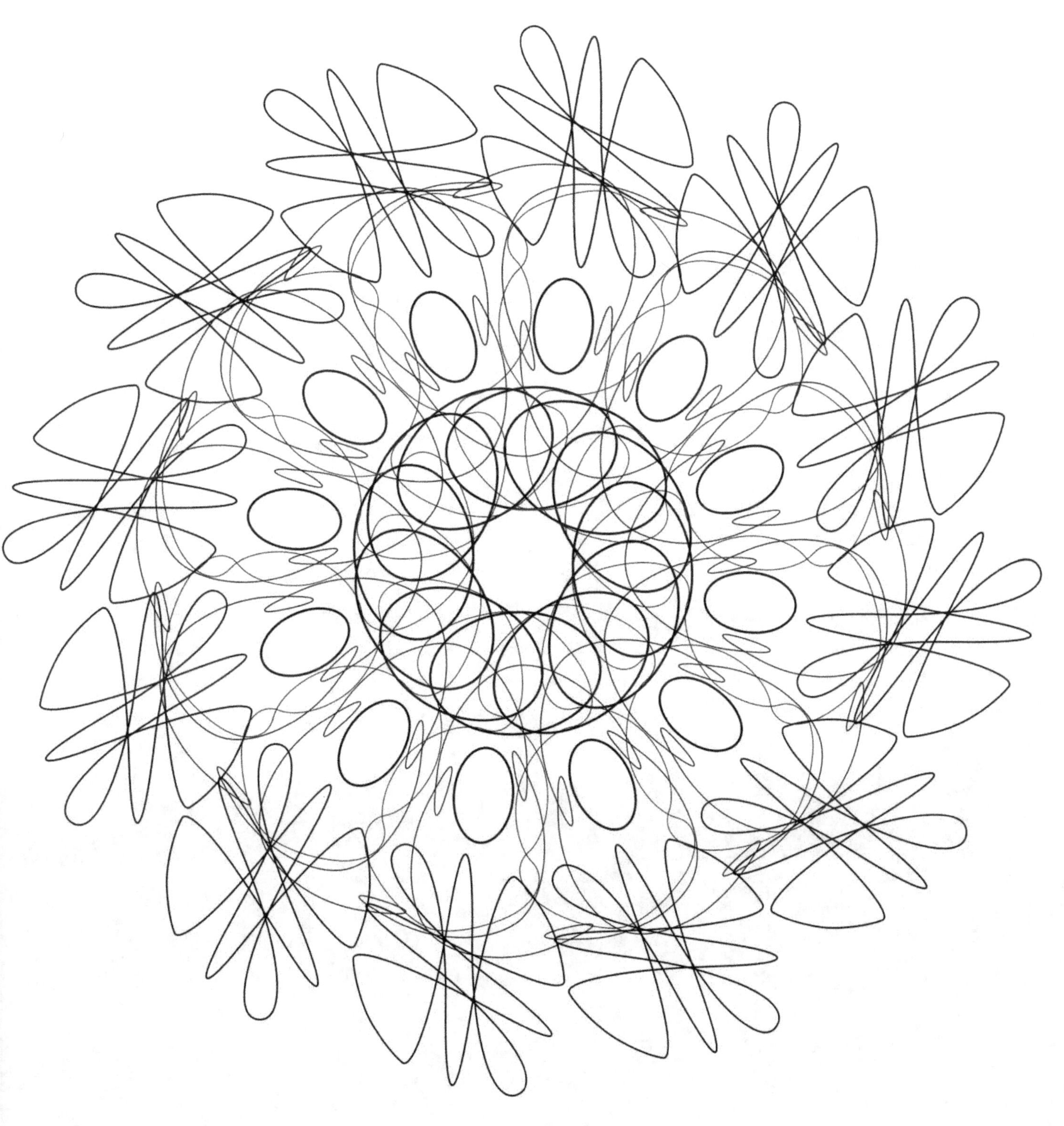

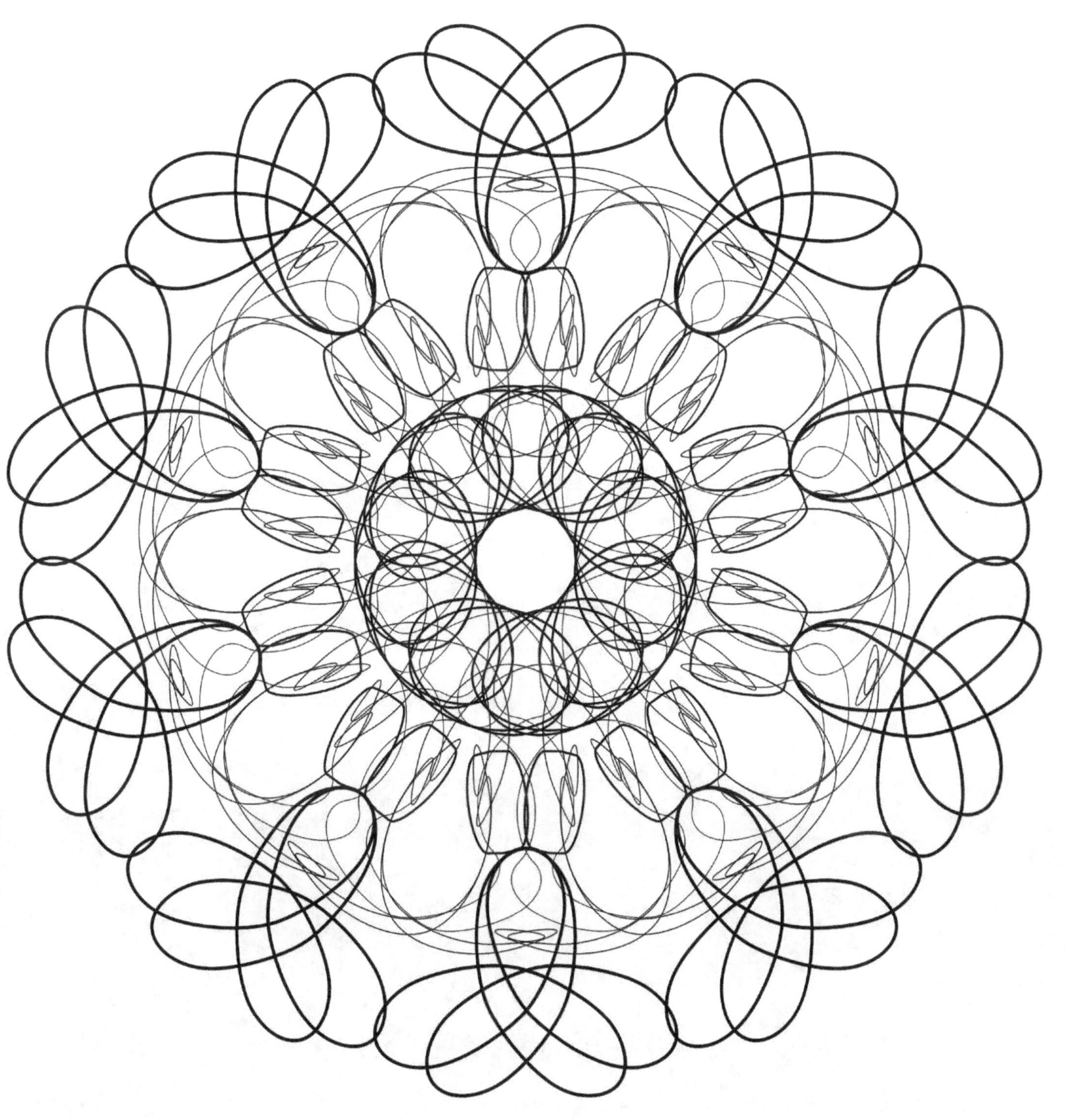

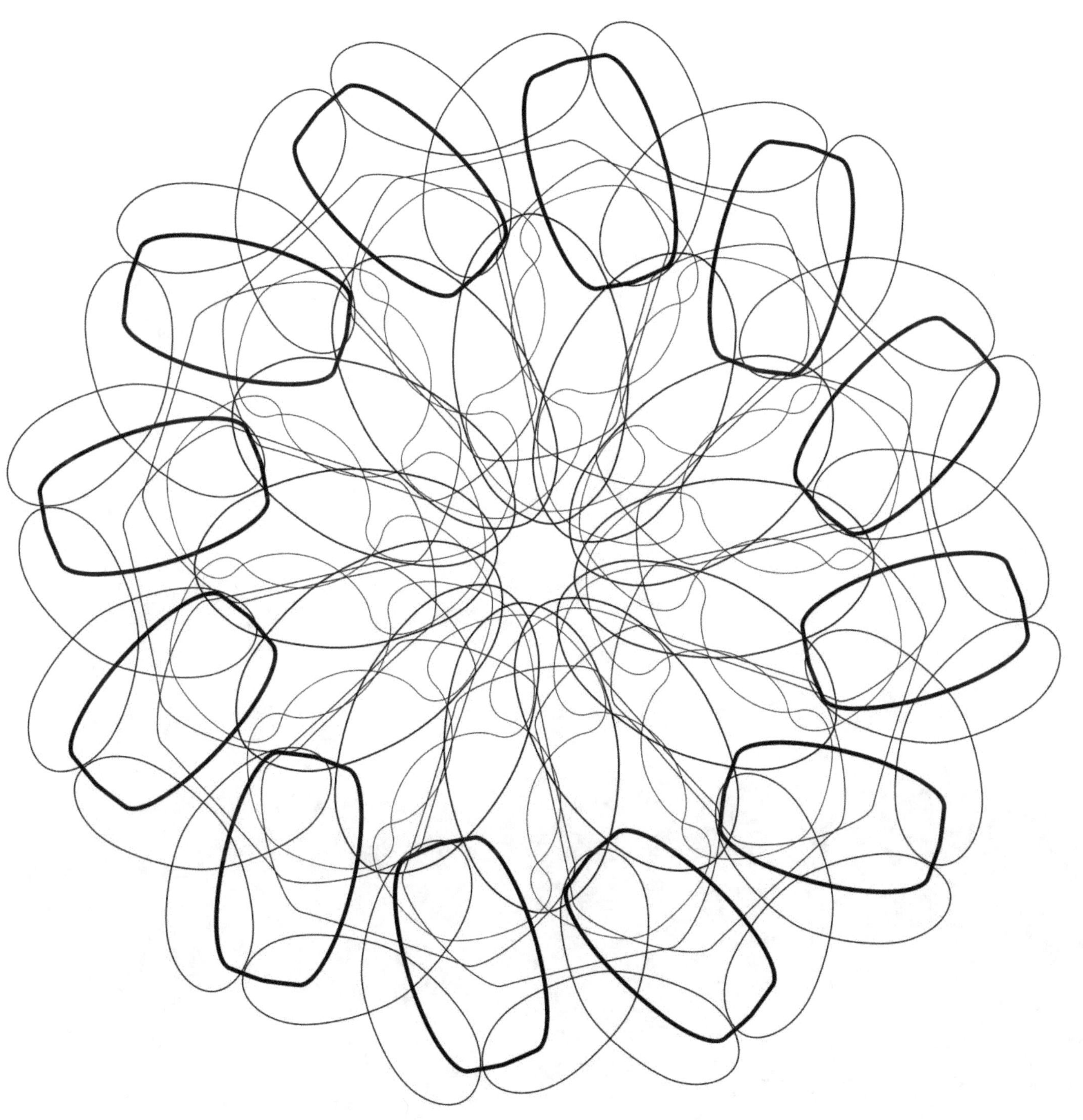

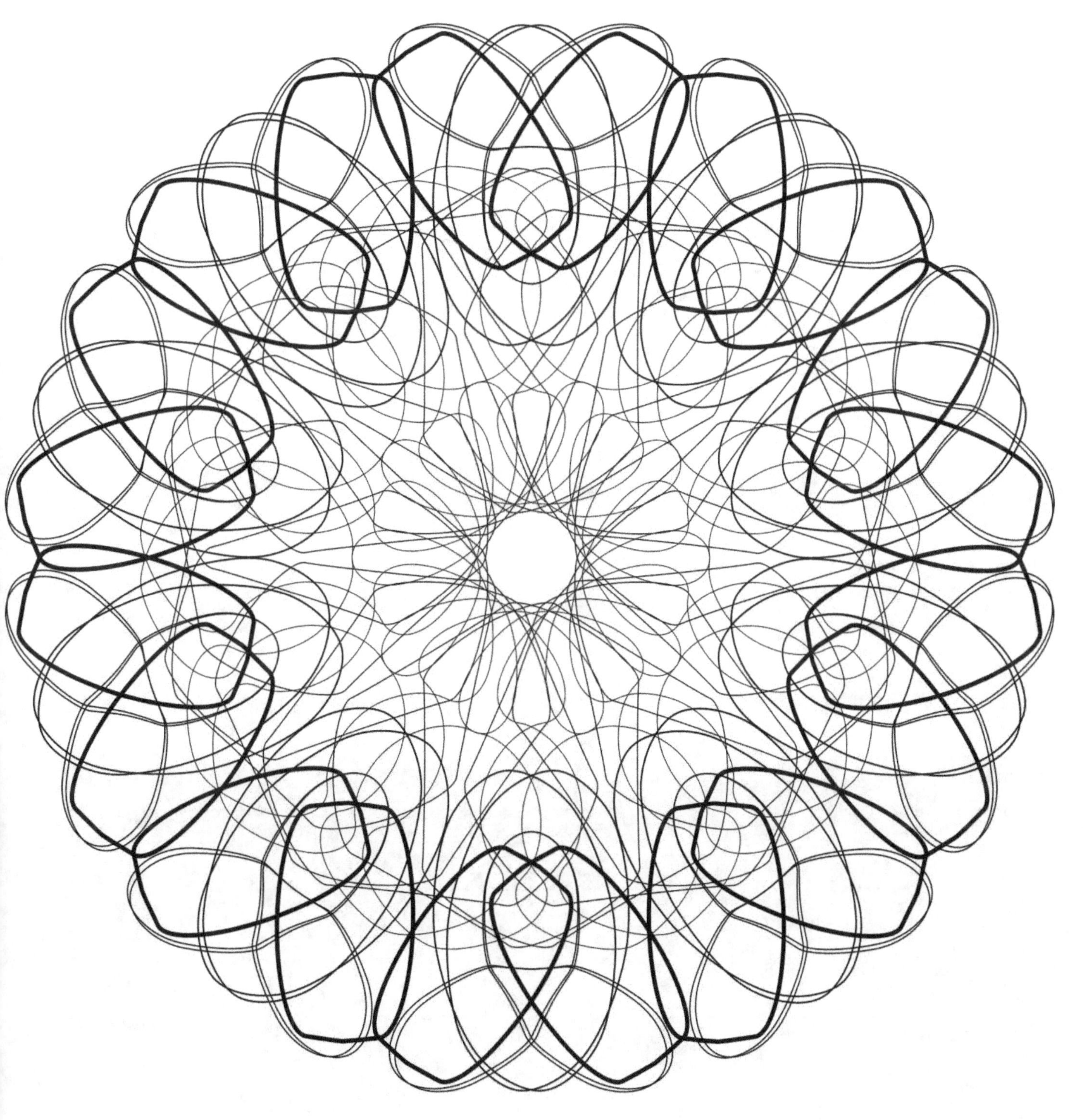

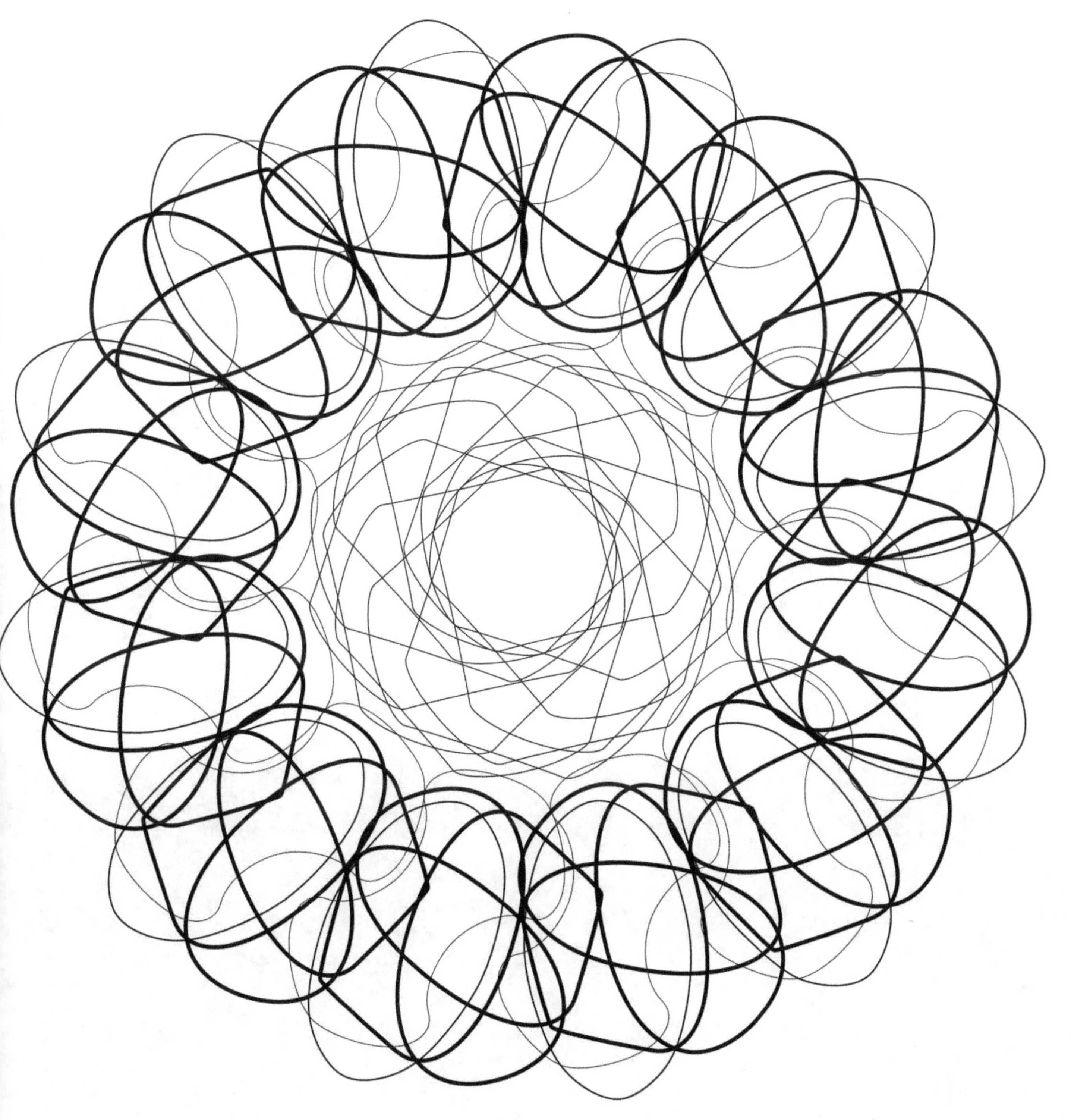

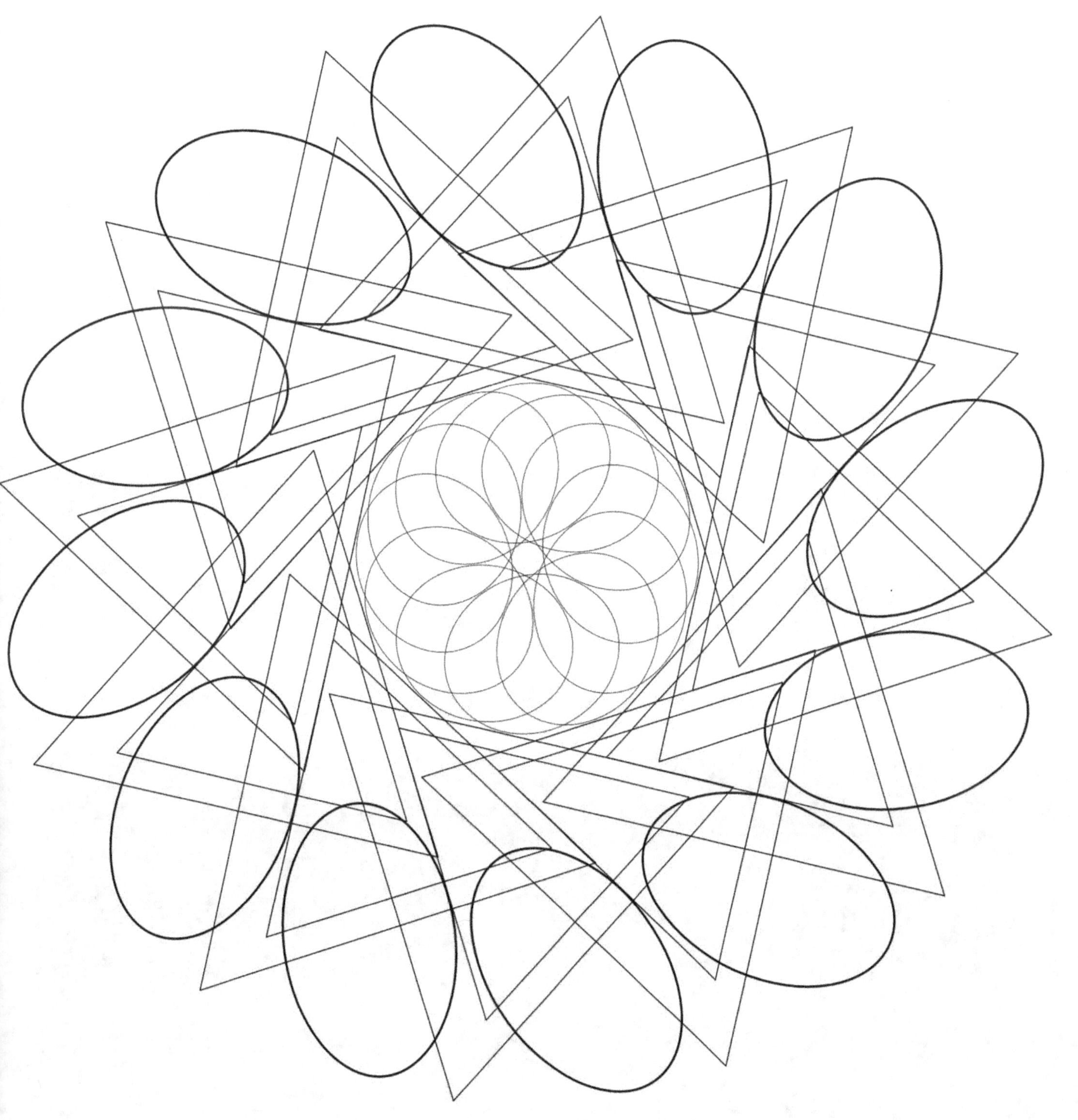

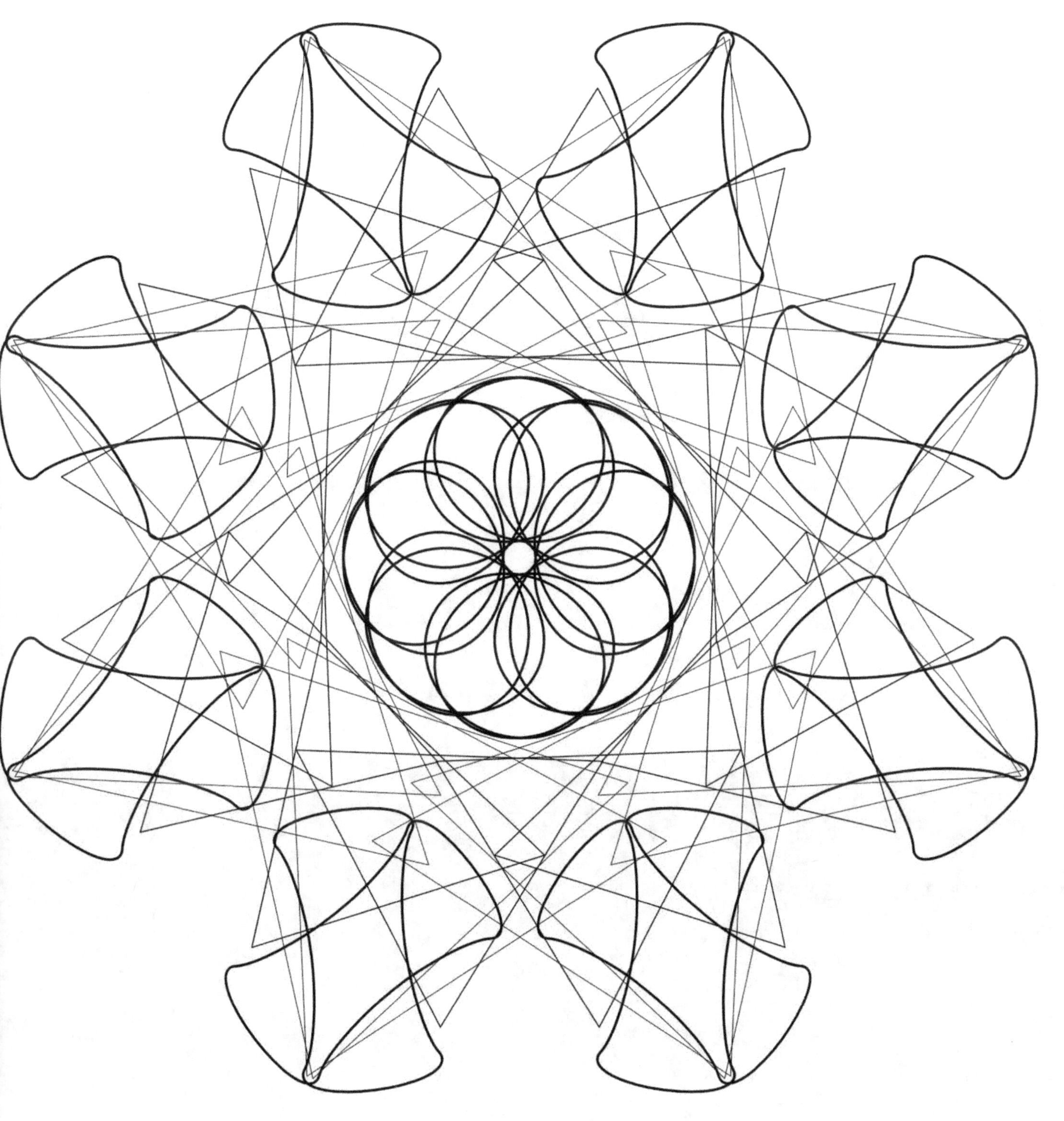

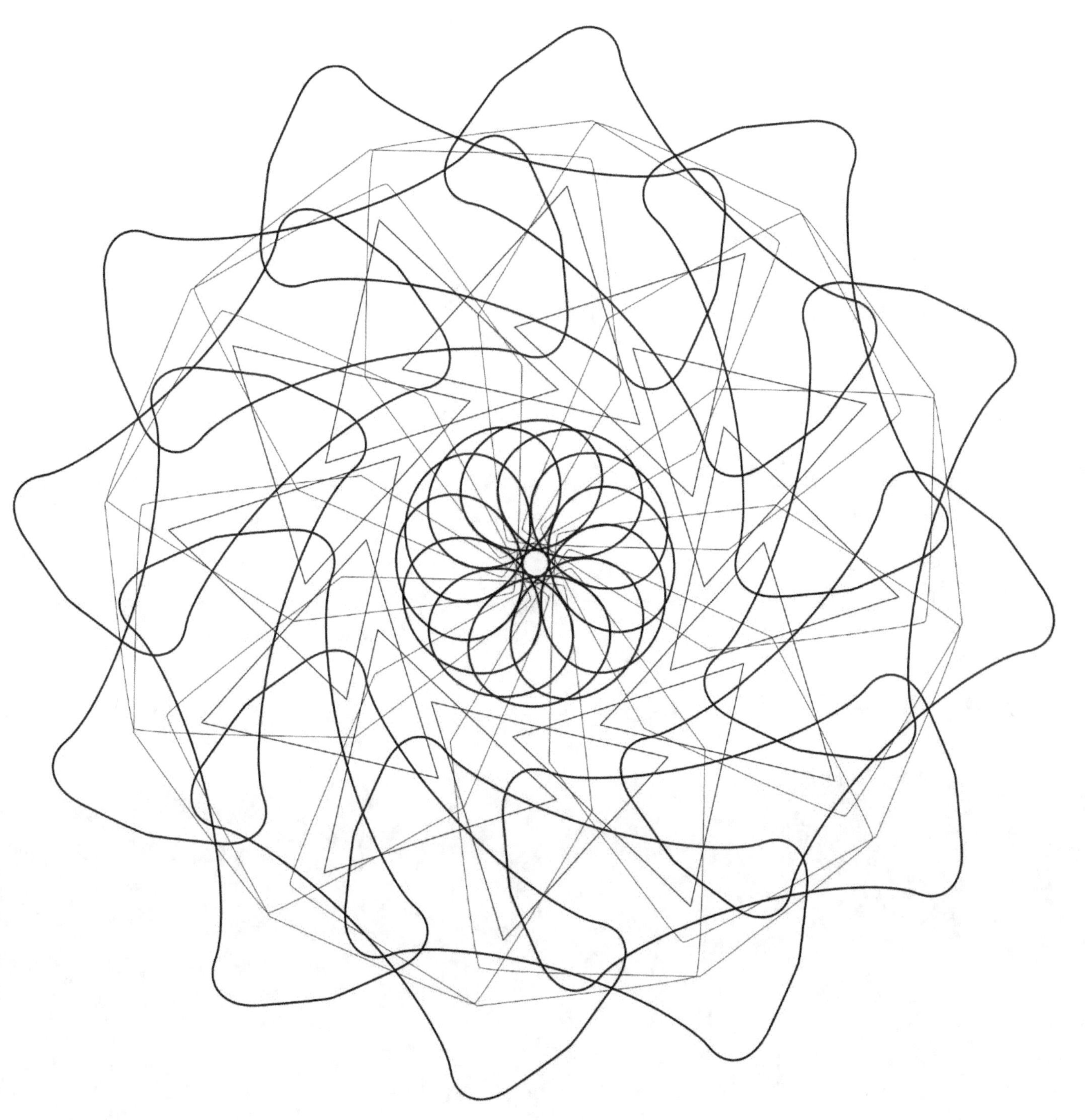

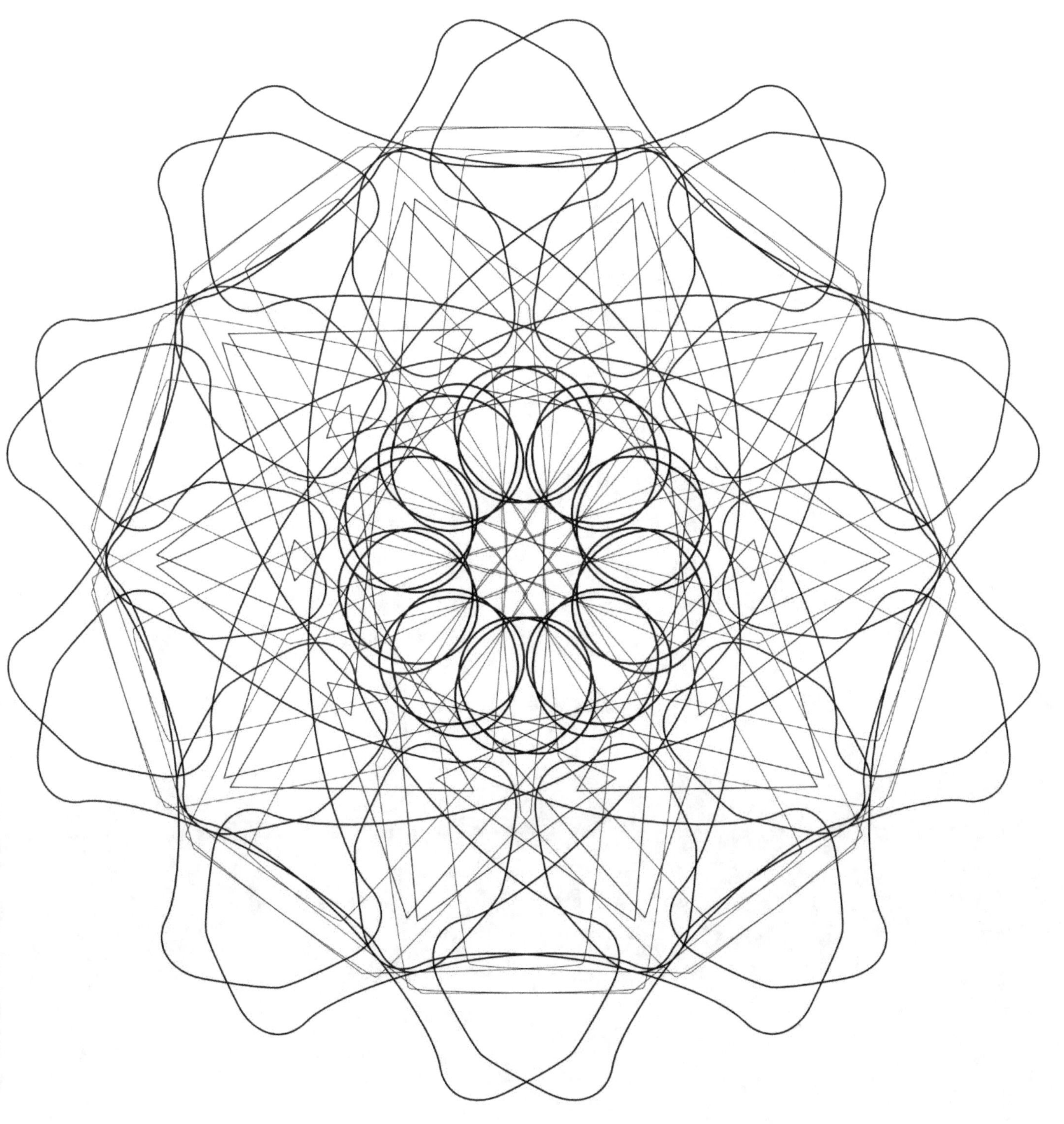

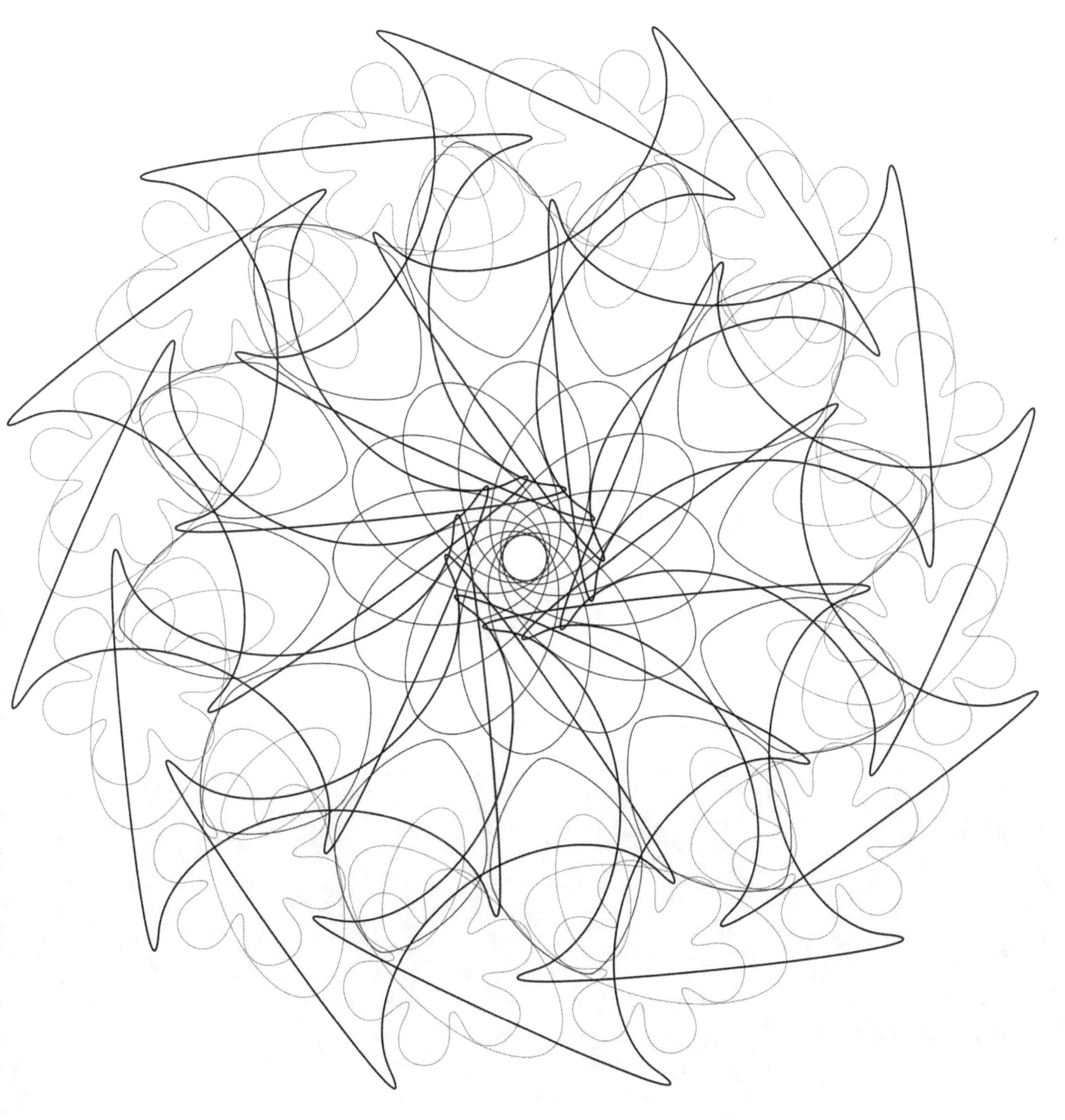

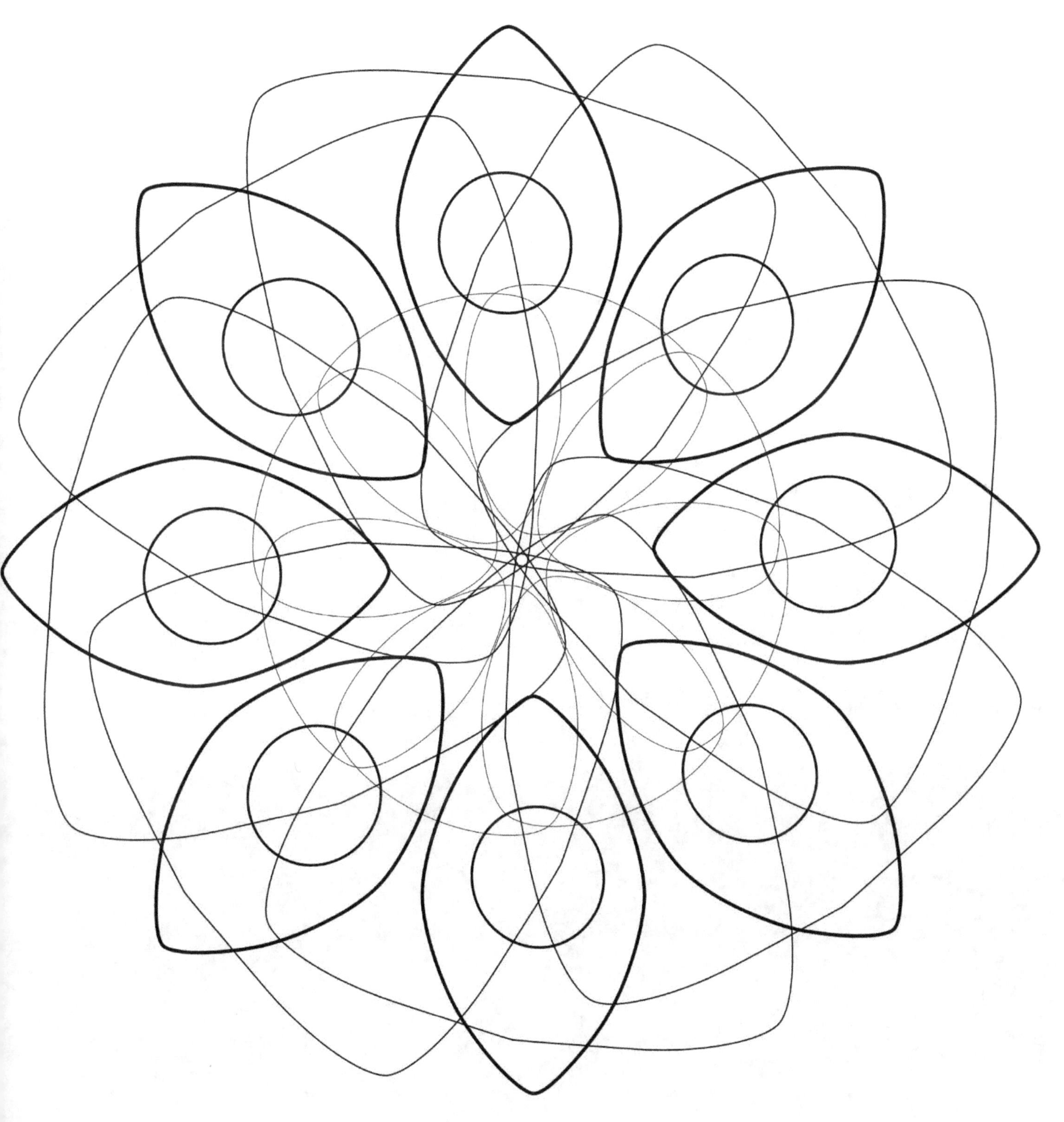

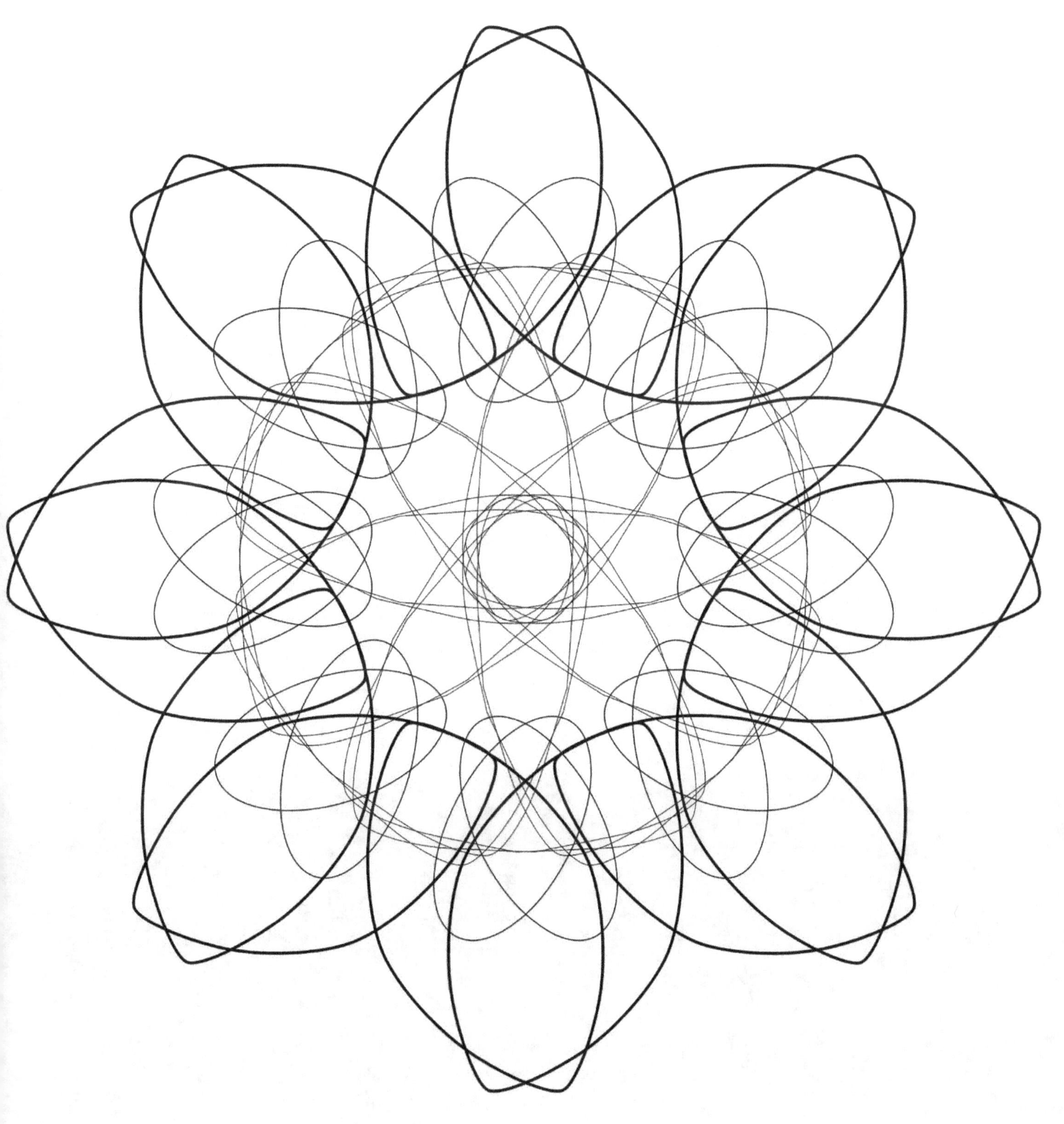

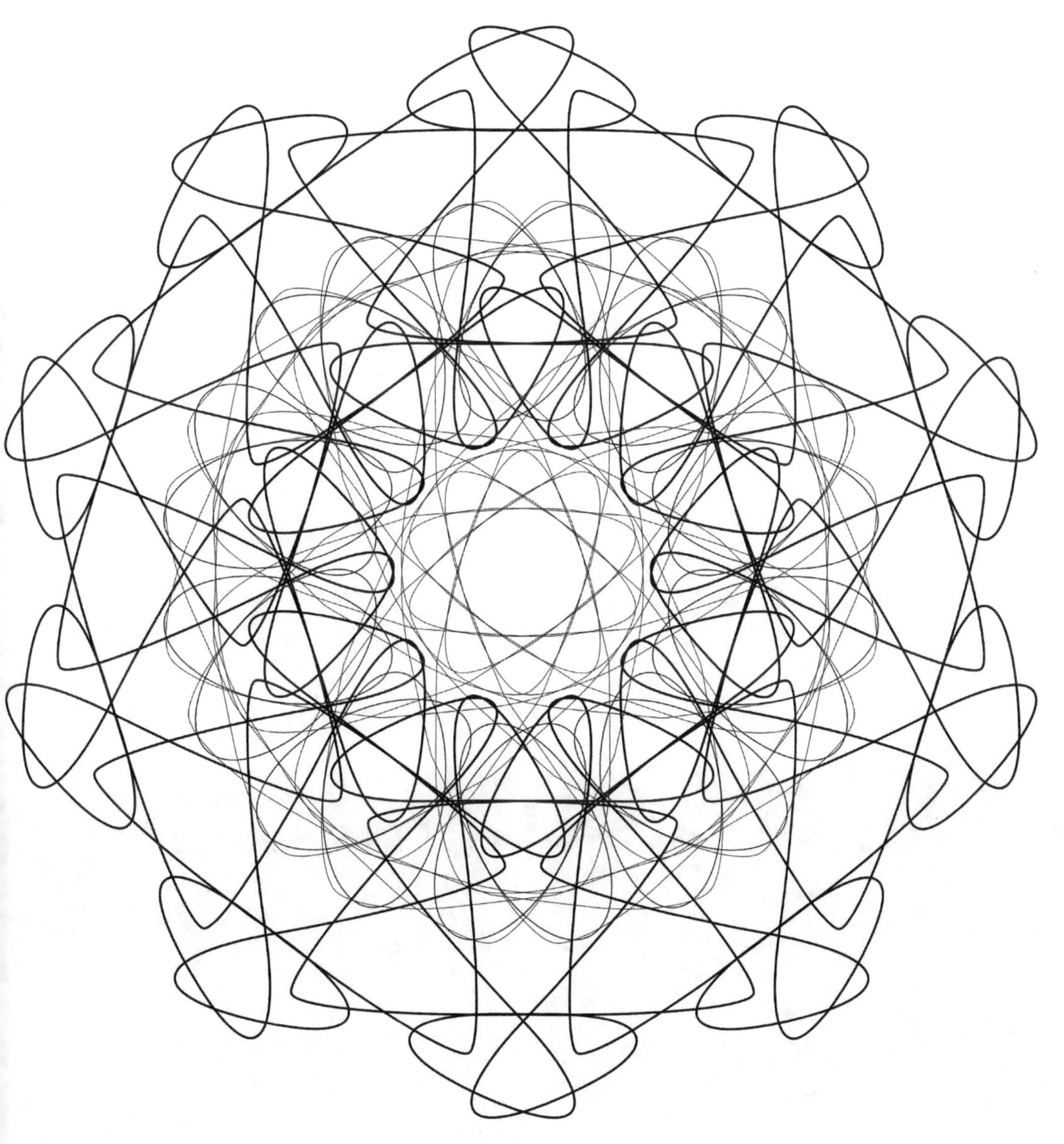

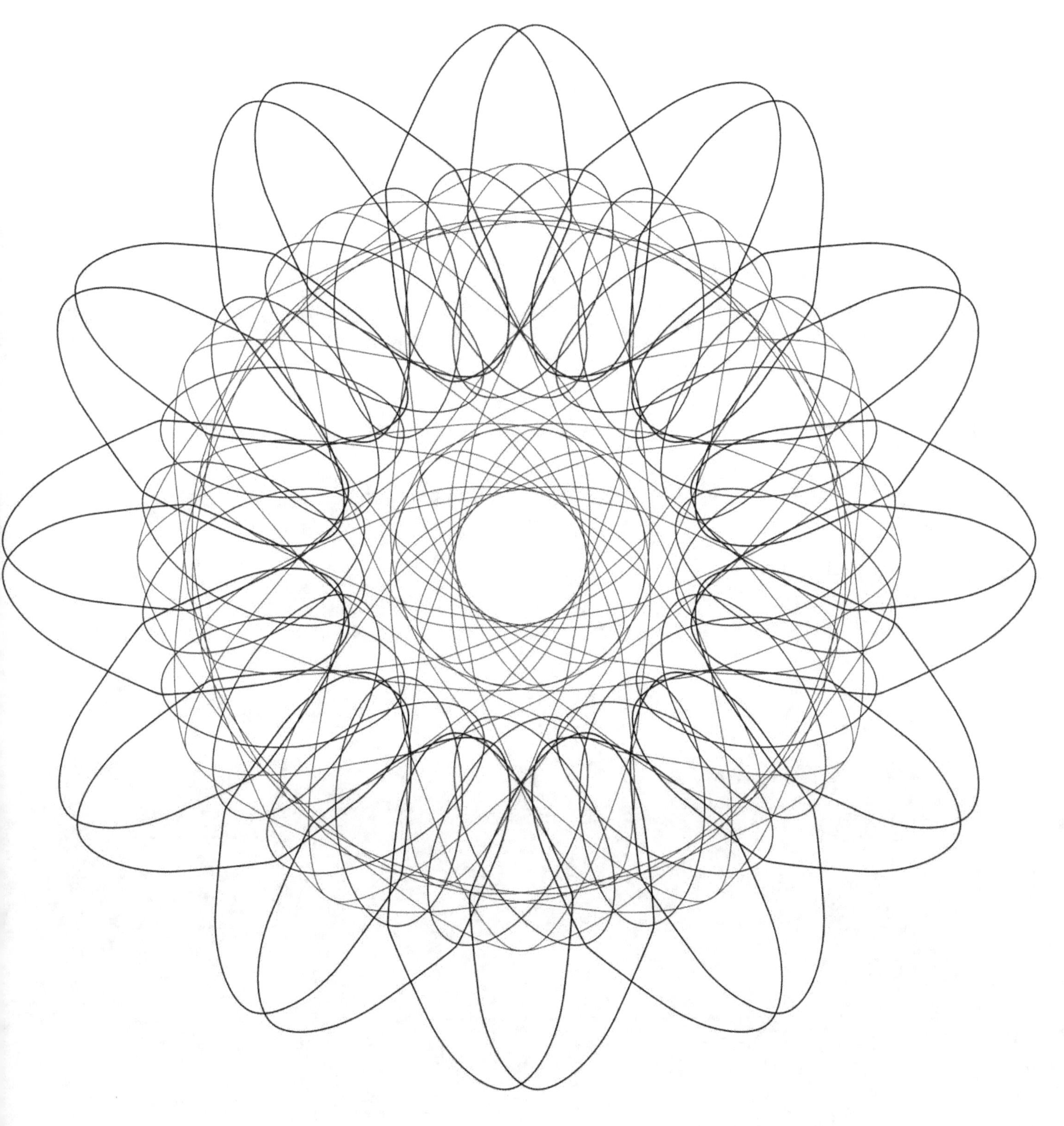

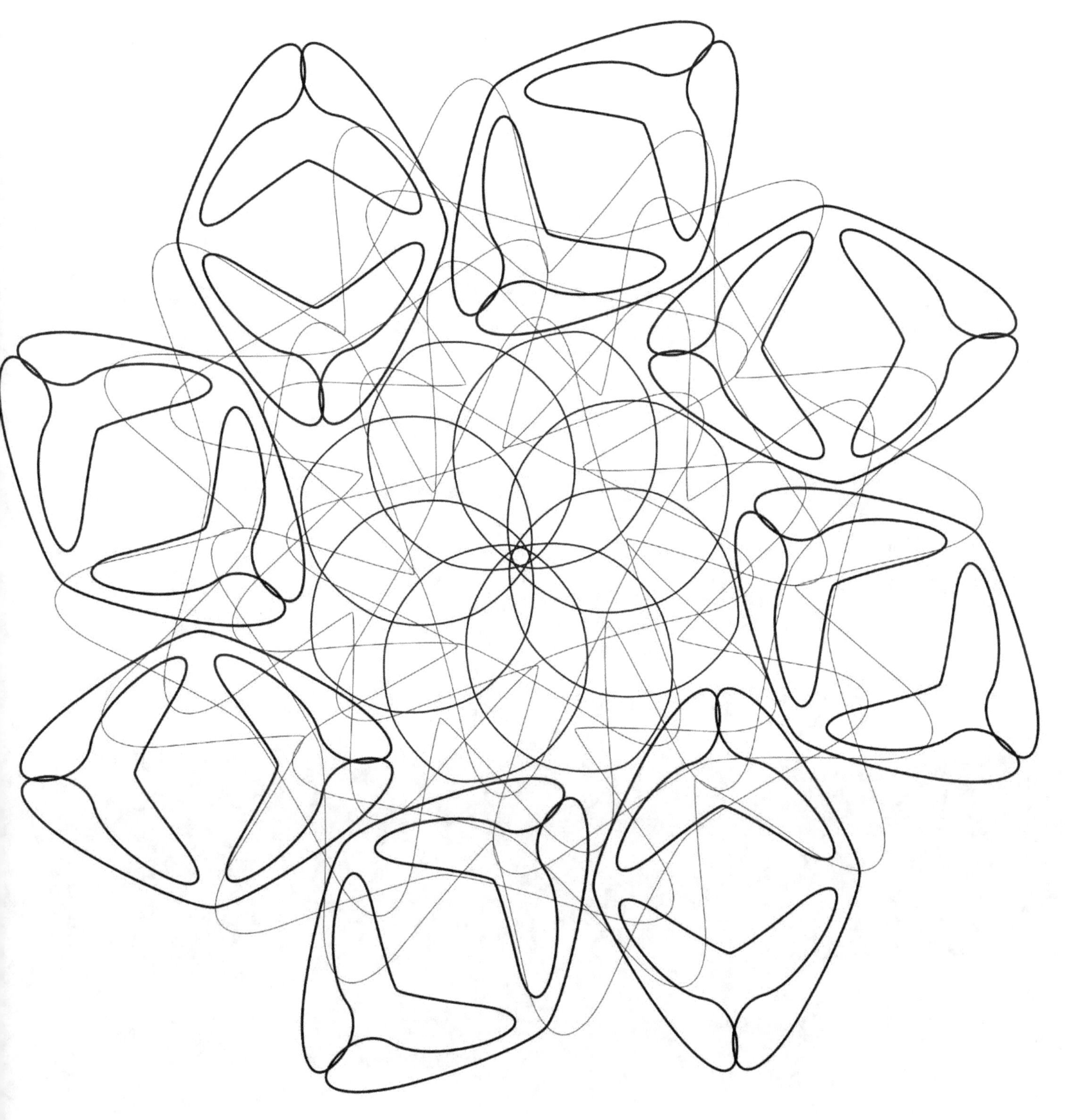

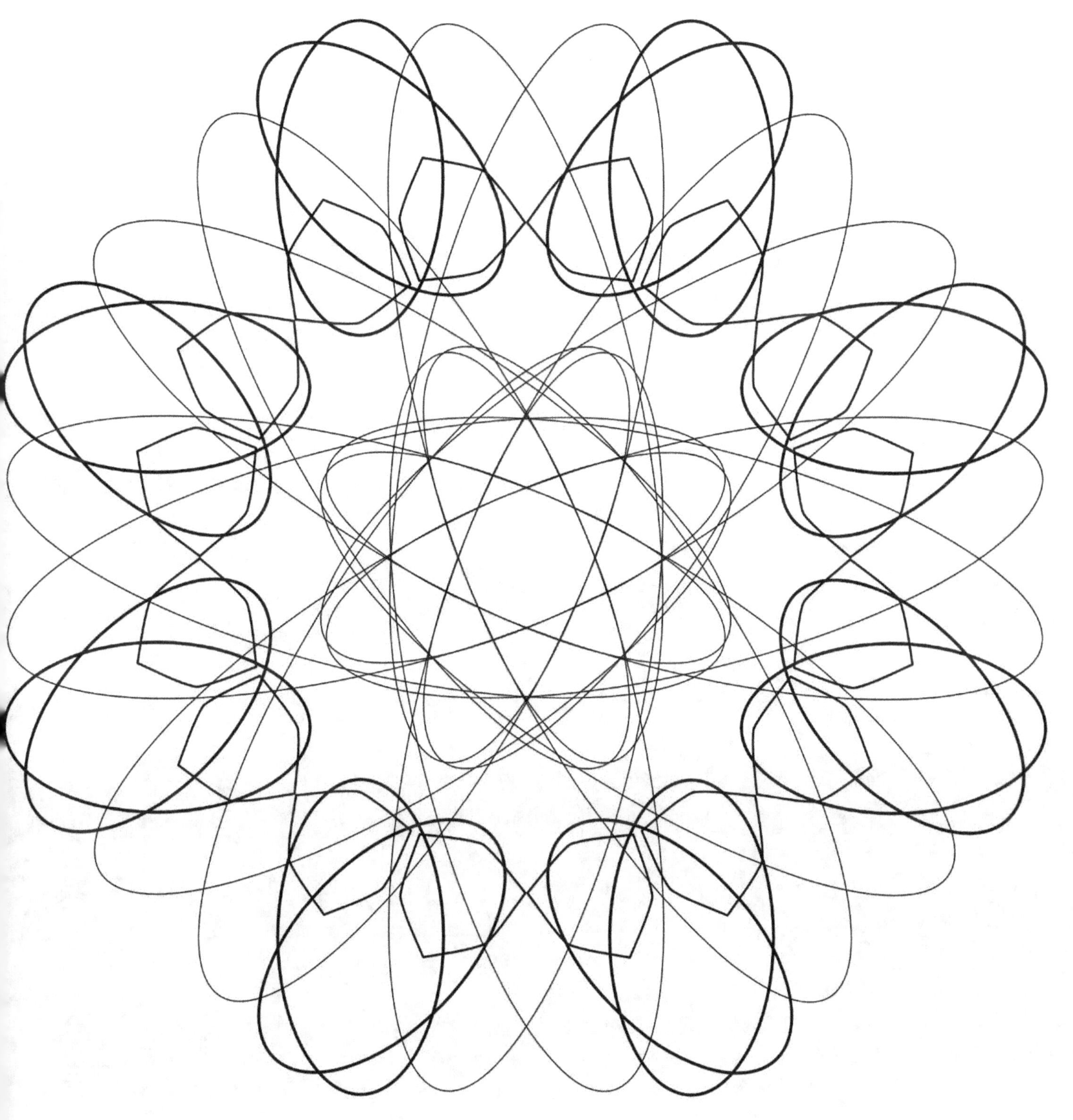

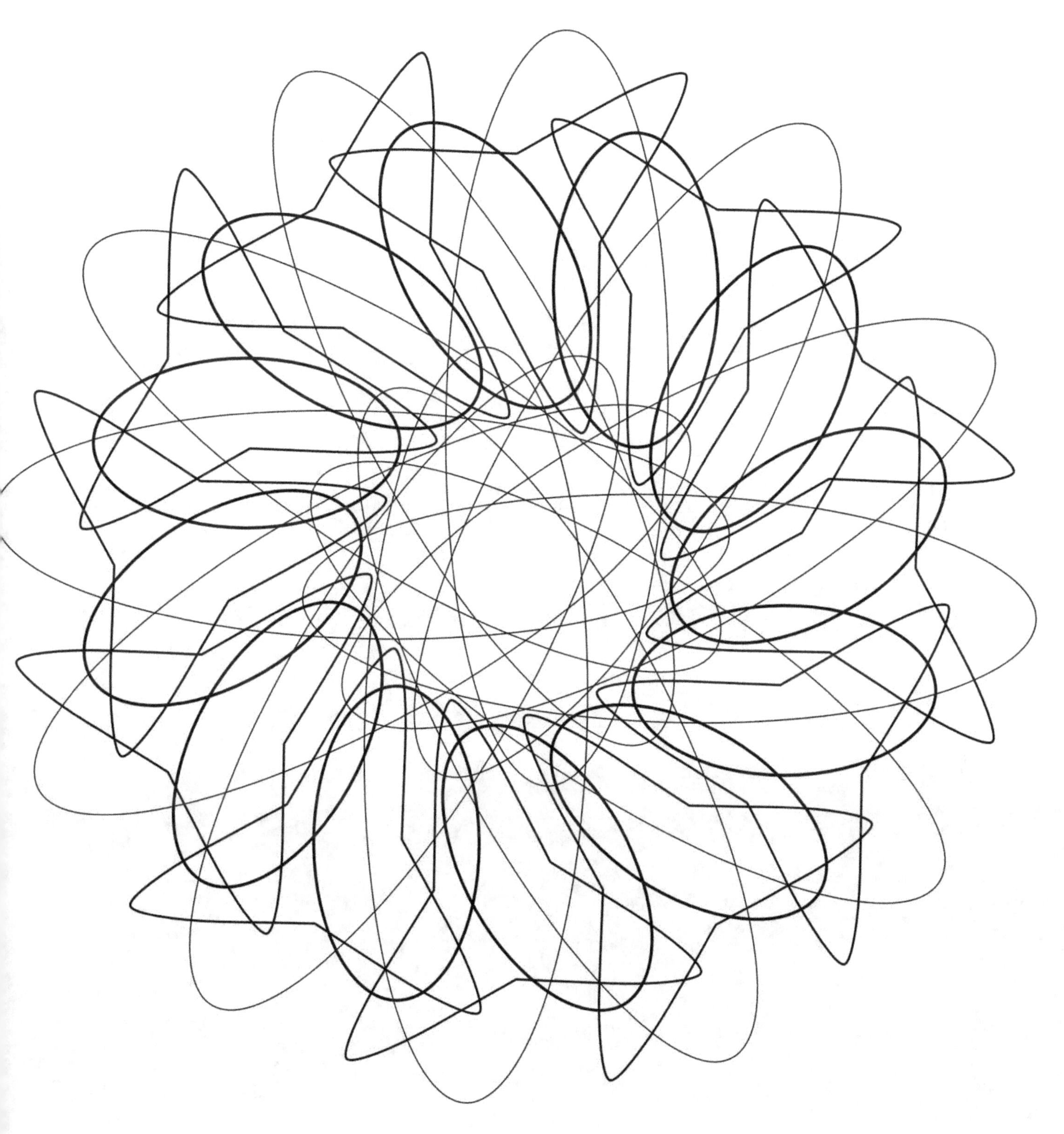

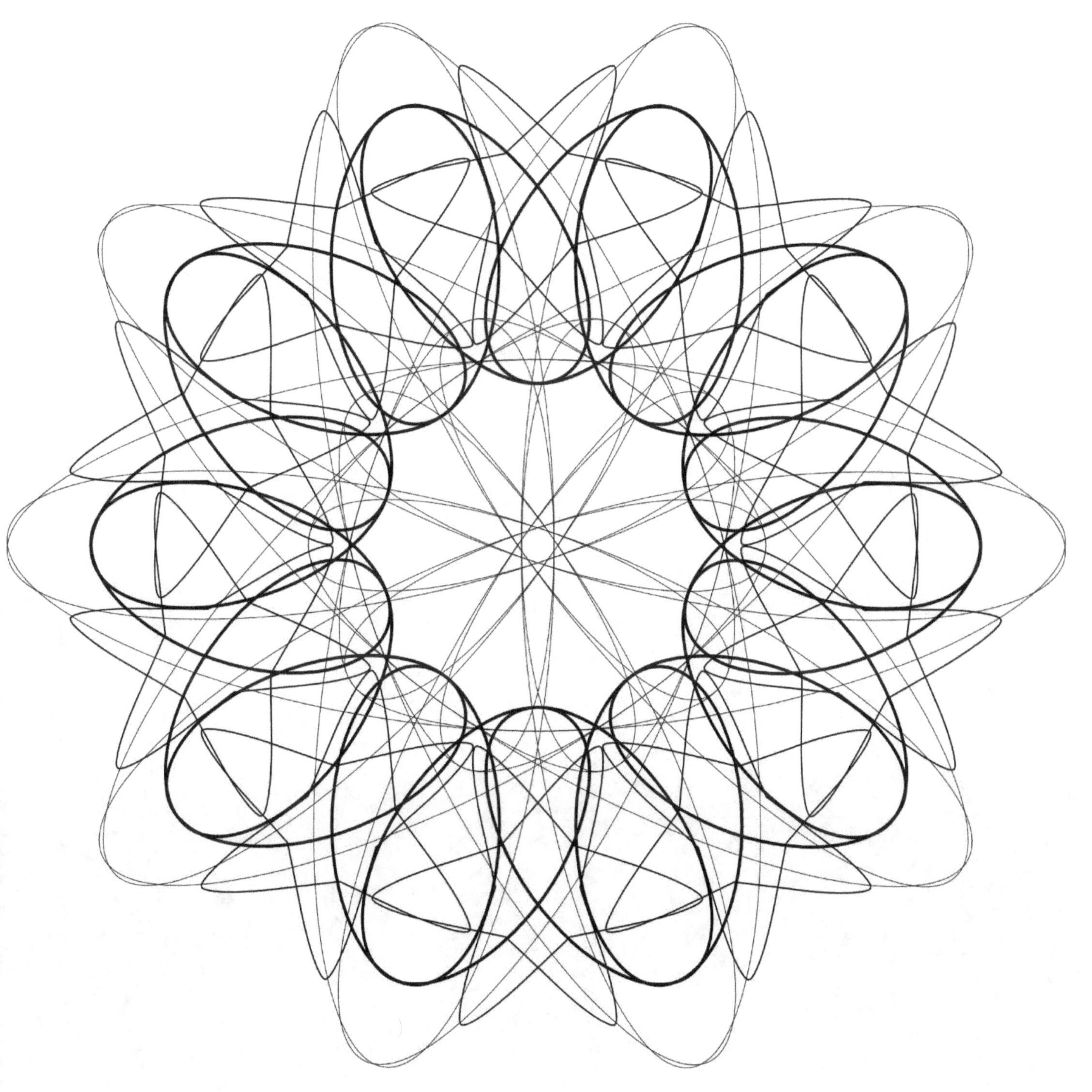

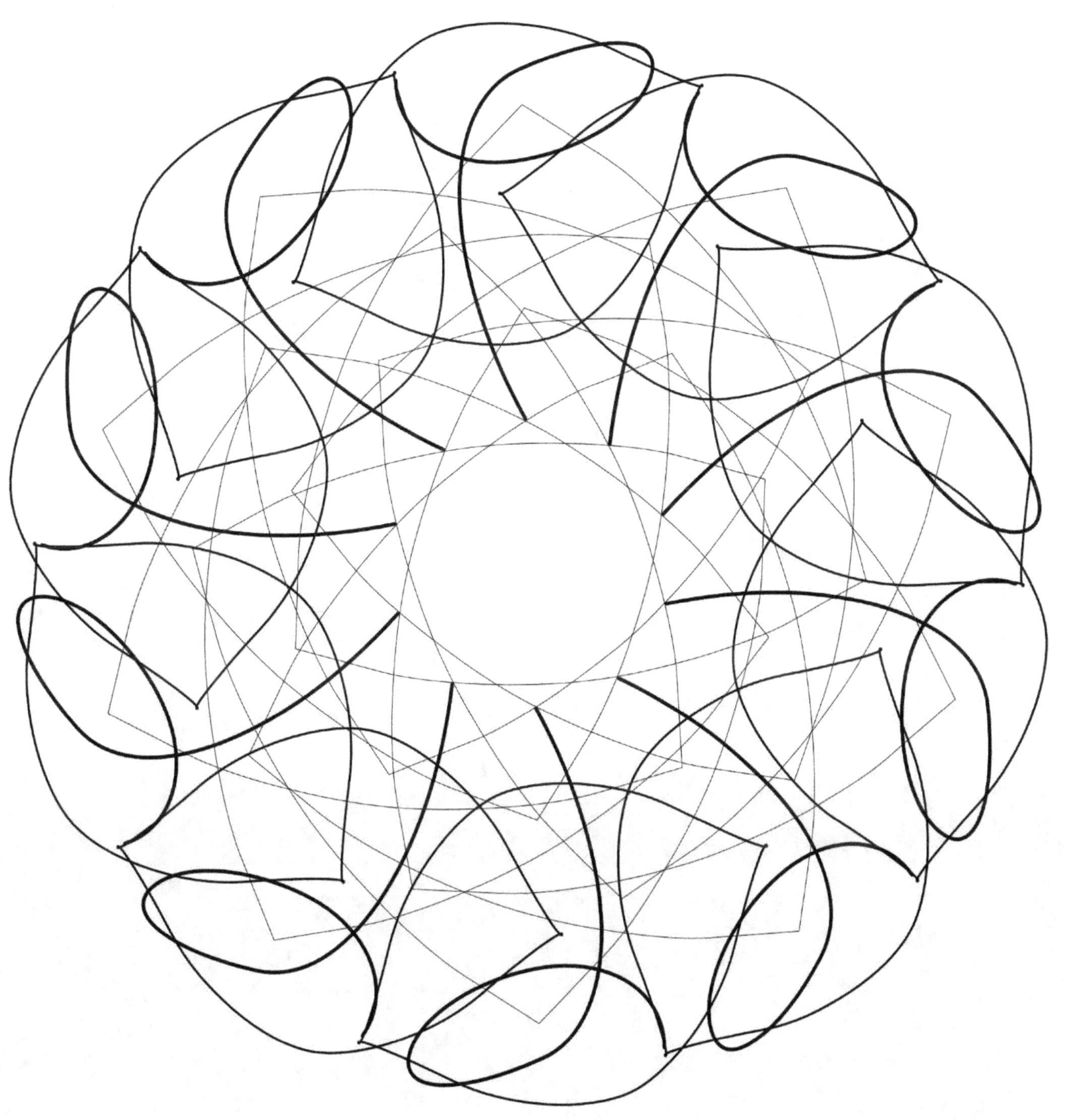

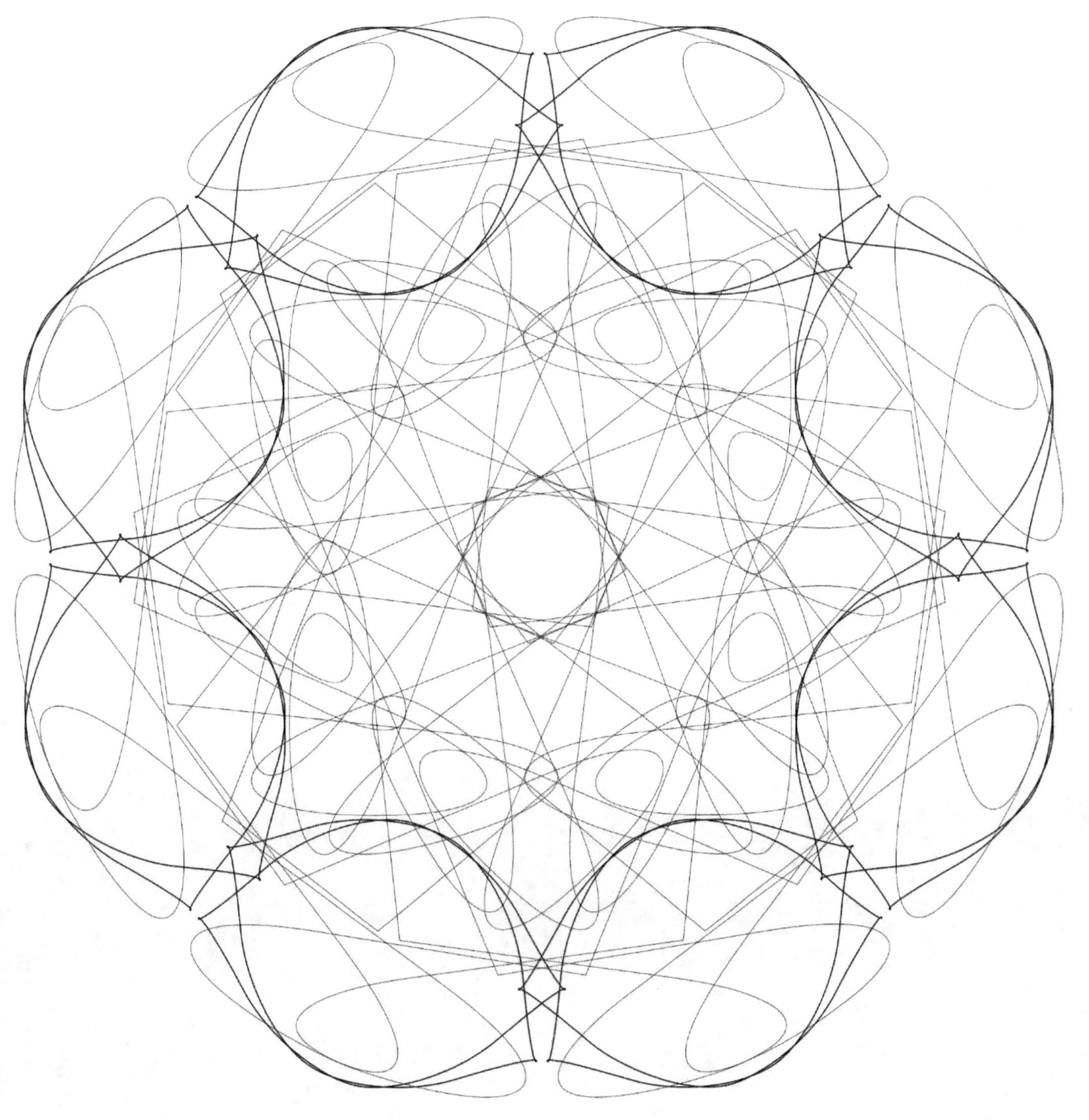

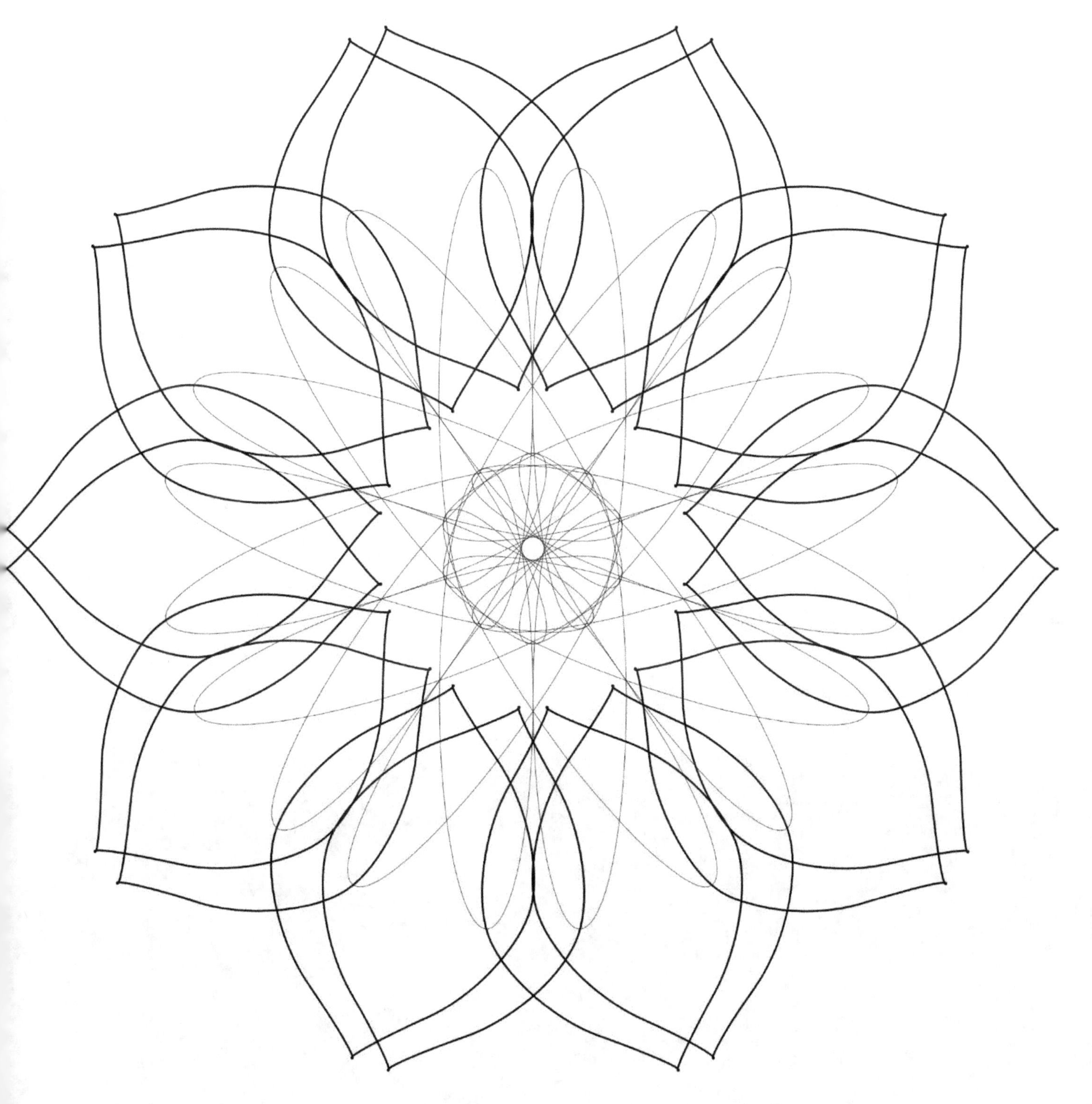

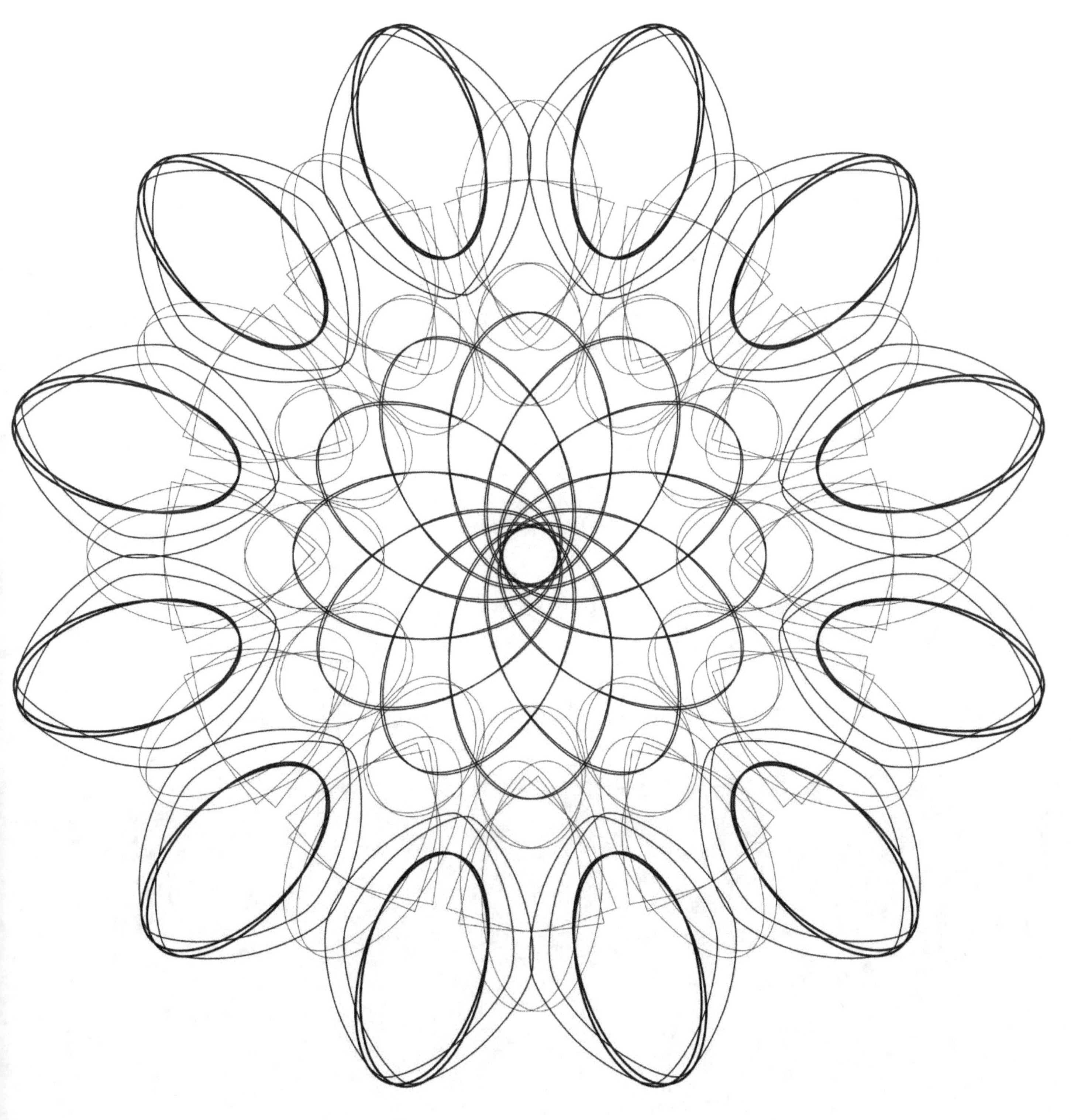

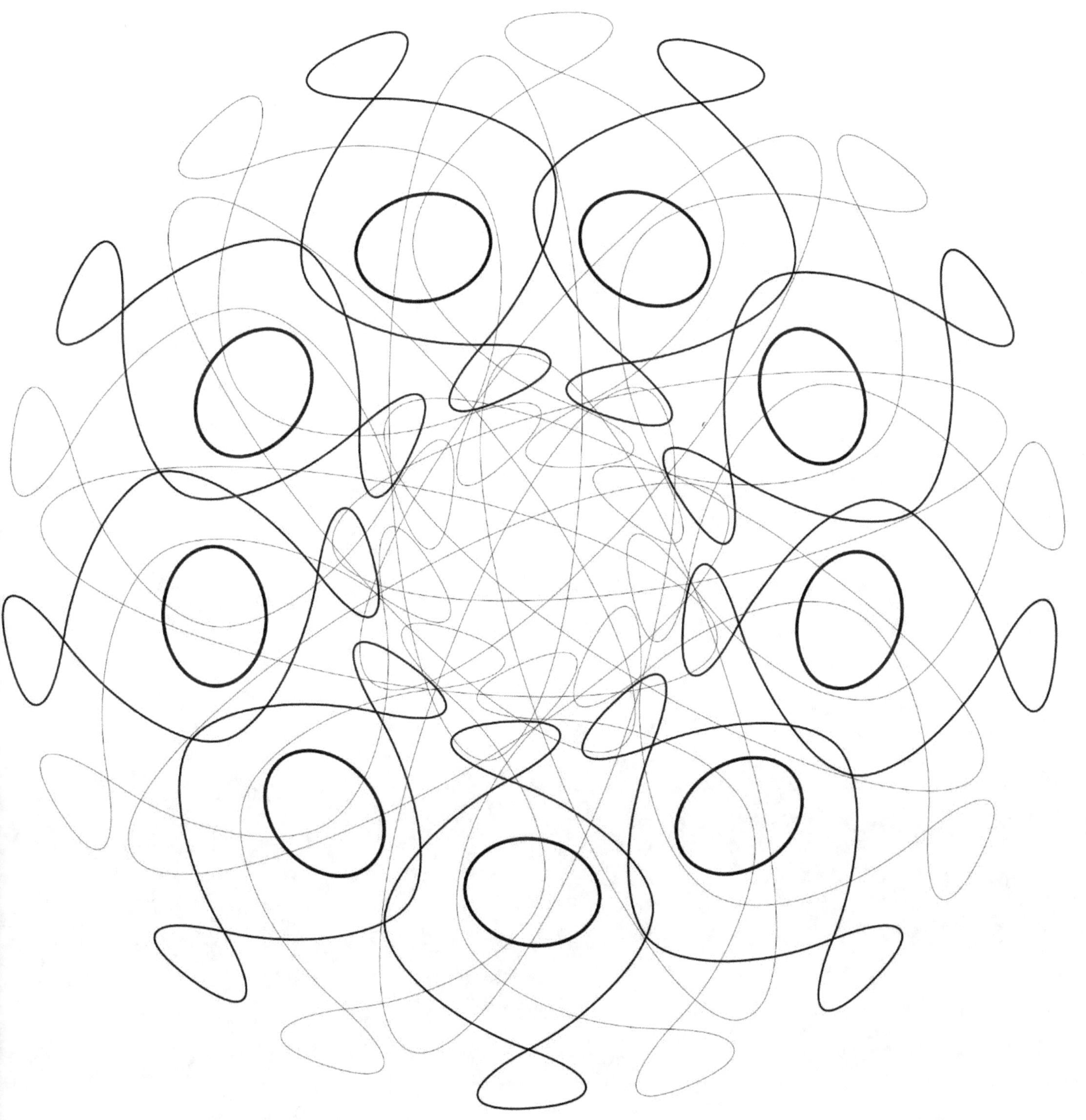

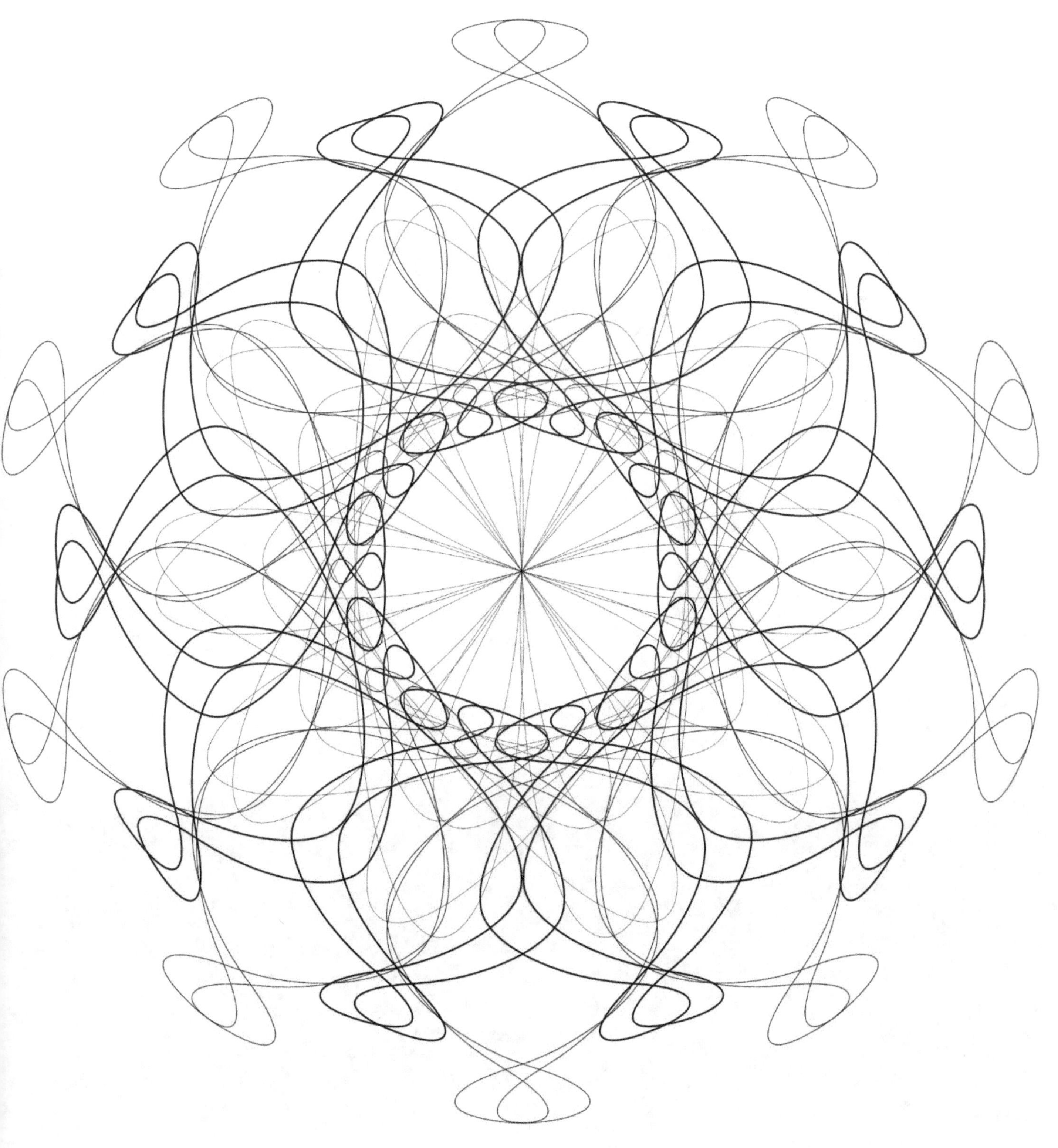

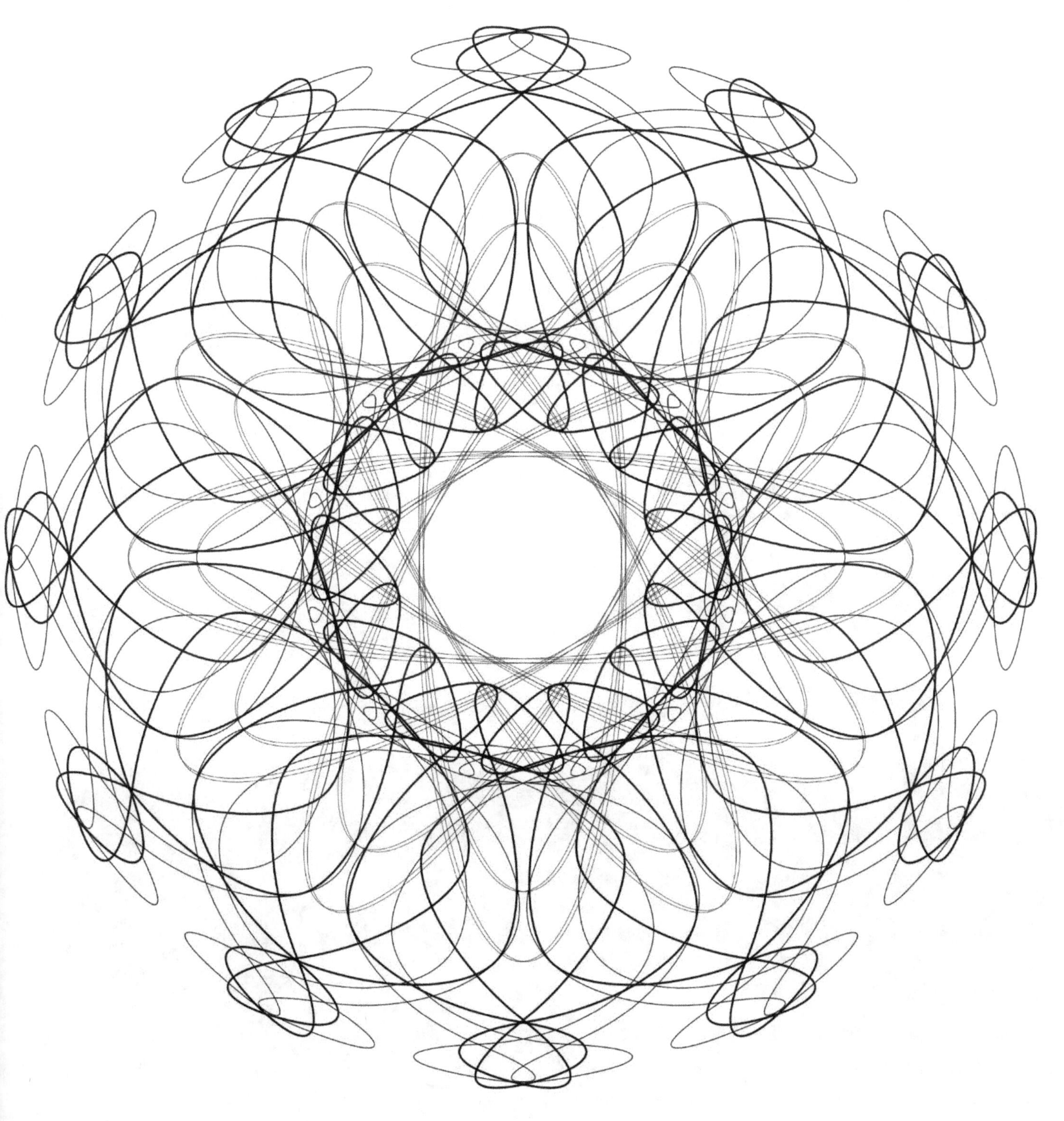

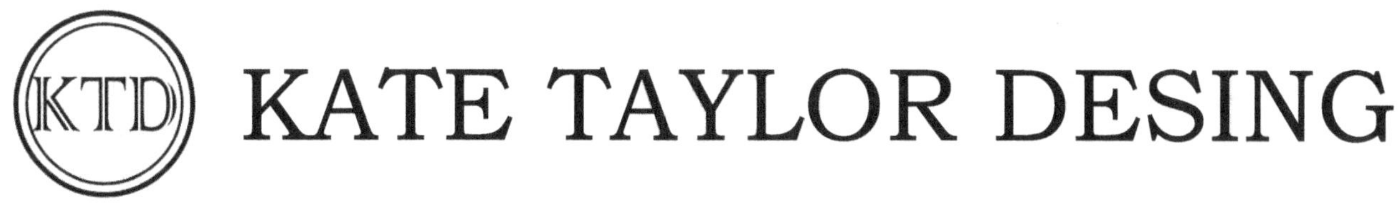

KATE TAYLOR DESING

OTHER COLORING BOOKS:

CARS

- American muscle cars coloring book for kids

- Supercars coloring book for kids

- Antique car coloring book for kids

- Jumbo cars coloring book for kids

MANDALAS AN PATTERNS

- Geometric shapes and patterns coloring book

- Adult coloring book tessellations patterns

- Adult coloring book geometric patterns

- Adult coloring book circular patterns.

- 150 Mandala coloring book

QUOTES

- Inspirational quotes from the bible coloring book

- Money quotes coloring book

- Quotes for success coloring book

- Funny Mom Quotes and Patterns coloring book

- Motivational swear words coloring book

HORROR

- Horror coloring book

www.ingramcontent.com/pod-product-compliance
Lightning Source LLC
Chambersburg PA
CBHW081727250726
48657CB00010B/3165